Neuroimaging - From Research to Clinical Practice

Edited by Sara Palermo

Published in London, United Kingdom

Neuroimaging - From Research to Clinical Practice
http://dx.doi.org/10.5772/intechopen.1005993
Edited by Sara Palermo

Contributors
Biyun Mo, Chiara Di Fazio, Derya Cayir, Fan Zhang, Jie Qin, Jing Ze Li, Lanxiang He, Lei Zhang, Mamoona Tariq, Maryam Afzaal, Naheed Akhter, Nur Aydinbelge Dizdar, Ping Yu, Sadia Sana, Sara Palermo, Tse Jung Liu, Wei Fu, WeiXia Chong, Xingyu Mu, Xinyuan Zhang, Yang Wu, Yasmin Mushtaq, Ye Wu, YuLong Zeng, ZuGuo Li

First published in London, United Kingdom, 2025 by IntechOpen
IntechOpen is the global imprint of INTECHOPEN LIMITED, registered in England and Wales, registration number: 11086078, 167-169 Great Portland Street, London, W1W 5PF, United Kingdom

For EU product safety concerns: IN TECH d.o.o., Prolaz Marije Krucifikse Kozulić 3, 51000 Rijeka, Croatia, info@intechopen.com or visit our website at intechopen.com.

British Library Cataloguing-in-Publication Data
A catalogue record for this book is available from the British Library

Neuroimaging - From Research to Clinical Practice
Edited by Sara Palermo
p. cm.
Print ISBN 978-1-83634-749-1
Online ISBN 978-1-83634-748-4
eBook (PDF) ISBN 978-1-83634-750-7

If disposing of this product, please recycle the paper responsibly.

Meet the editor

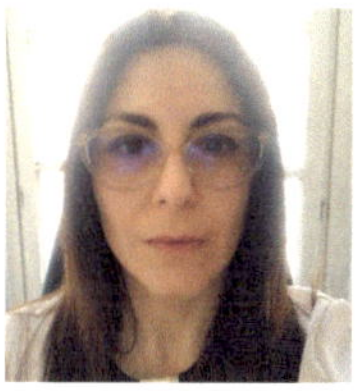

Sara Palermo holds an MSc in Clinical Psychology and a Ph.D. in Experimental Neuroscience. She is an Associate Professor of Neuropsychology and Cognitive Neuroscience at the University of Turin, where she teaches in the Master's program in Body and Mind Sciences and the School of Specialization in Neuropsychology. A member of the Neuroscience Institute in Turin, she also consults for the Neuroradiology Department at IRCCS Istituto Neurologico. She is affiliated with several national and international societies, including the APA, SINdem, AIP, and the European Academy of Neurology. As an emerging researcher, she is building expertise in neuroimaging, contributing to understanding brain disorders and ageing.

Contents

Preface

Over the past few years, neuroimaging has increasingly assumed a central position within the neuroscientific and medical community, moving from being a tool for research analysis to a real lever of daily clinical application. This book, *Neuroimaging – From Research to Clinical Practice*, was conceived to accompany the reader along this path, illustrating the necessary steps, from looking at developing brain to clinical diagnosis and therapeutic and surgical application guided by images.

The text is divided into three main sections, each covering a specific area of neuroimaging in current times, to provide an expansive yet solid view of the subject, lending credibility to the recent technological advances and their actual impact on patient treatment. The book's latter part covers neuroimaging's impact on neurological and psychiatric disease diagnosis and treatment. With functional and multimodal approaches, imaging turns into an invaluable associate of the physician, increasing diagnostic accuracy and delineation of therapeutic strategies.

The volume starts with a chapter dedicated to one of neuroscience research's most difficult and fascinating challenges: understanding brain development during the first years of life. In "Advanced Diffusion MRI in the Developing Brain", the potential of diffusion magnetic resonance imaging (dMRI) to shed light on pediatric brain microstructure is explored. In clear but somber writing, the authors illustrate how sophisticated imaging techniques allow us to track early changes in the brain during life, with significant implications for the diagnosis and early therapy of neurodevelopmental disorders.

The second part of the book addresses the influence of neuroimaging in the diagnosis and treatment of neurological and psychiatric diseases. Thanks to functional and multimodal techniques, imaging has become a standard tool for the physician, improving diagnostic accuracy and the individuation of therapeutic strategies. The chapter "Connection between Diseases and Neuroimaging of the Nervous System" offers an integrative clinical-radiological reading model of neurological disease, highlighting the correlation of clinical observations, imaging data, and diagnosis. This contribution is aimed particularly at clinicians who desire to enhance their interpretative skills with a systemic and practice-oriented approach. This is then followed by "Functional Neuroimaging in Nuclear Medicine", where the application of nuclear medicine in dementia, movement disorders, and drug-resistant epilepsy is discussed. The authors explain how these techniques, even in the most complex cases, facilitate accurate localization of the brain areas.

Finally, "Clinical Applications of PET/CT in Neuroimaging: Case-Based Approach" gives a real-life overview through real clinical cases to show how PET/CT makes possible the identification of metabolic and functional alterations in neurodegenerative disorders, epilepsy, and brain tumors.

The third and final section introduces the reader to an extremely cutting-edge field of practice: employing advanced neuroimaging to guide surgical and therapeutic treatments. In these chapters, the image becomes not merely an instrument of observation, but an active portal between doctor, patient, and brain. In the chapter "Interventional Neuroimaging: Techniques, Applications, and Future Directions", the third and final section introduces the reader to an extremely cutting-edge field of practice: employing advanced neuroimaging as a guide to surgical and therapeutic treatments. In these chapters, the image becomes not merely an instrument of observation, but an active portal between doctor, patient, and brain. The volume is rounded out with the contribution "Neuronavigation: Neuroimaging Applied to Neuromodulation and Neurosurgery", where neuroimaging applications in brain surgery and neuromodulation (e.g., DBS and TMS) are detailed. Because the structural and functional imaging can now be combined, neuronavigation facilitates more precise, safer, and less invasive interventions. The authors also provide a glimpse of things to come in the field, with references to augmented reality, point-of-care imaging, and machine learning in the operating room.

Together, these chapters witness a period of great excitement over neuroimaging as the convergence of research, technology, and clinical practice brings new opportunities for diagnosing and treating nervous system disorders. *Neuroimaging – From Research to Clinical Practice* is hoping to serve as a handbook and source of information for experts and researchers interested in learning about how the science of pictures is transforming the boundaries of modern medicine.

Sara Palermo
Department of Psychology,
Neuroscience Institute of Turin,
University of Turin,
Turin, Italy

Section 1

Advanced Techniques and Brain Development

Chapter 1

Advanced Diffusion MRI in Developing Brain

Ye Wu, Lanxiang He, Xinyuan Zhang and Fan Zhang

Abstract

Brain development takes a long time, starting in the third trimester of pregnancy and continuing into the first decade of life. Understanding how the brain develops in early life is important for identifying abnormal development that may later be related to neurological and psychiatric disorders. Diffusion MRI (dMRI) is a powerful imaging technique that shows how water molecules move in biological tissues, providing important information about brain tissue structure and organization. Although dMRI has shown significant advances in pediatric research over the last 30 years, the study of early brain development is still relatively new but has great scientific and clinical potential. This chapter assesses how advanced dMRI methods can be used to measure rapid and dynamic changes in the microstructural foundations of the brain during early life.

Keywords: brain, development, dMRI, microstructure, connectome

1. Introduction

The development of the brain is affected by genetic, environmental, and physiological factors and is crucial for the examination of neurodevelopmental disorders and cognitive functions. Advances in neuroimaging, bioinformatics, and experimental models have offered valuable insights, including the Adolescent Brain Cognitive Development (ABCD) Study, which aims to understand how environmental factors influence the development of adolescents' behaviors and brains with a multimodality neuroimaging dataset. In particular, dMRI is a powerful imaging technique that uses the movement of water molecules to gain detailed insight into the microscopic structure of biological tissues [1]. In biological tissues, the motion of water is restricted by cellular elements such as cell membranes, myelin sheaths, and cytoskeletons. By assessing the direction and extent of water diffusion, dMRI can infer the alignment and integrity of these elements [2].

In recent years, there has been growing interest in the relationship between brain development and the connectome, especially with advances in dMRI data from the Lifespan Human Connectome Project [3] and the ABCD study. These data have provided valuable information on brain organization and potential structural changes that occur during adolescence, the genetic impact on brain connectivity, and the link between brain connectivity, cognitive function, and psychopathology. Furthermore,

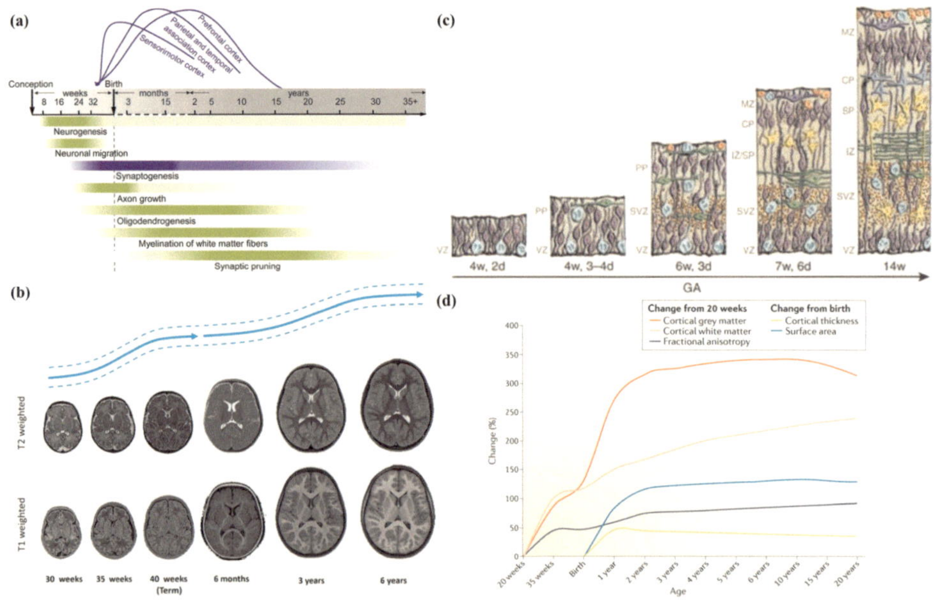

Figure 1.
The intricate processes involved in human brain development. (a) The maturational processes of the human brain, encompass neurogenesis, synaptic pruning, myelination, and other critical developmental stages. (a) Adapted from: Ref. [5]. (b) T1- and T2-weighted images at different age points during the perinatal and early childhood period, accompanied by growth curves. (b) Adapted from: Refs. [6–8]. (c) The schematic illustration of the embryonic layers of the developing human neocortex. (c) Adapted from: Refs. [9, 10]. (d) The estimated trajectories of brain structural parameters during development. (d) Adapted from: Refs. [11, 12].

research has explored how the structural connectome of human white matter is connected to the neuronal and cellular architecture of the brain [4], collectively enhancing our understanding of the evolving connectome and its implications for neurodevelopmental outcomes.

As a noninvasive technique, dMRI enables researchers and medical professionals to examine the composition and integrity of white matter pathways, which are crucial for efficient neural connections. Widely used to study brain development in children and adolescents and age-related degenerative processes, dMRI helps to understand typical developmental patterns while identifying early signs of neurodevelopmental disorders (**Figure 1**). Its broad applications in neuroscience and medicine include exploring brain development and aging and understanding and diagnosing various neurological and psychiatric disorders [13]. Despite the challenges they pose, ongoing advancements in dMRI technologies and methods show promising potential to improve our understanding of the brain and improve clinical outcomes.

2. Advanced diffusion MRI techniques

2.1 High angular resolution diffusion imaging (HARDI)

With dMRI, diffusion tensor imaging (DTI) [1] was introduced in the mid-1990s and has since become essential to study the integrity and organization of white matter in the brain and other tissues. DTI relies on the anisotropic movement of water in fibrous tissues, such as the white matter of the brain [14], where water molecules are more likely to move along the lengths of axons than across them due to the constraining influence of cell membranes and myelin sheaths [15]. Although DTI has greatly improved our understanding of white matter, its inability to precisely differentiate crossing fibers within a voxel. Unlike DTI, HARDI, an advanced dMRI method [16], enables the reconstruction of complex white matter pathways by collecting diffusion data in a much larger number of directions, providing enhanced connectivity mapping, which is crucial to understanding communication and interactions between different regions of the brain.

2.2 Diffusion kurtosis imaging (DKI)

DKI is an improvement in HARDI that goes beyond traditional methods such as DTI [17]. Structural barriers in biological tissues obstruct water diffusion, resulting in non-Gaussian diffusion patterns. Unlike DTI, which assumes a Gaussian distribution (**Figure 2(a,b)**), DKI captures the non-Gaussian behavior of water diffusion in biological tissues, providing more comprehensive insights into the microenvironment, especially in complex tissue regions. DKI measures the kurtosis of the diffusion signal to quantify these deviations. High kurtosis values indicate complex and restricted diffusion environments, while low kurtosis values suggest simpler, less restricted diffusion. Changes in kurtosis metrics during brain development may reflect the maturation of neural pathways and the increasing complexity of brain tissue. The ability of DKI to capture non-Gaussian diffusion makes it more sensitive to subtle changes in tissue microstructure than DTI [21].

2.3 Neurite orientation dispersion and density imaging (NODDI)

NODDI is an advanced dMRI method designed to provide comprehensive information on the complex microstructural makeup of brain tissues [22]. NODDI was developed to measure the density and dispersion of neurites, including axons and dendrites (**Figure 2(c,d)**). NODDI overcomes the limitations of conventional dMRI methods by using a multicompartmental modeling approach to analyze the diffusion

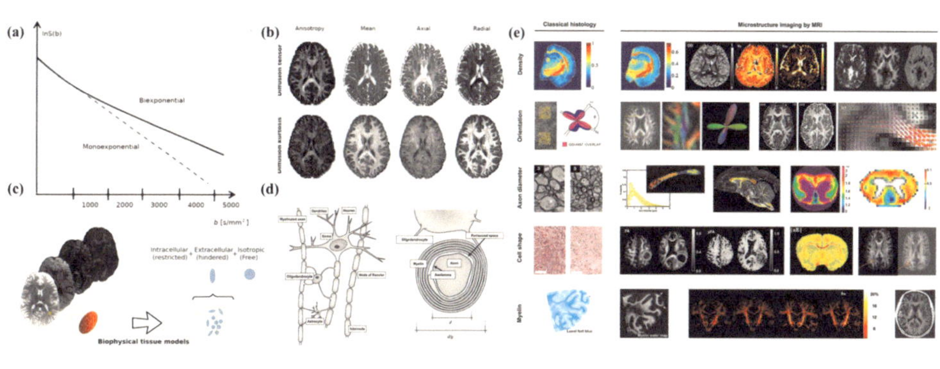

Figure 2.
(a) The dMRI signal decay at higher b values illustrates non-Gaussian diffusion, particularly in two-compartment systems like white matter (WM), leading to a bi-exponential signal decay. (b) Scalar DTI and DKI maps are exemplified, (c) alongside an overview of biophysical tissue microstructure models, highlighting intra-axonal (restricted), extra-axonal (hindered), and CSF (free, isotropic water) diffusion compartments. (a–c) Adapted from: Ref. [18] (d) The cellular composition of brain tissue, with a focus on neurons and glial cells. (d) Adapted from: Ref. [19]. (e) A comparison is made between classical histology and microstructure imaging techniques, showcasing various techniques organized by target tissue feature. (e) Adapted from: Ref. [20].

signal, thus differentiating between different tissue components and providing more detailed microstructural information. Derived from NODDI, the neurite density index (NDI) measures the percentage of tissue volume occupied by neurites. Higher NDI values indicate an increase in neurite density, often associated with healthy and well-organized brain tissue. The Orientation Dispersion Index (ODI) measures the variability in neurite orientation. Higher ODI values indicate more complex and dispersed neurite orientations, potentially indicating the presence of intricate neural networks. The Isotropic Volume Fraction (fiso) evaluates the proportion of tissue volume taken up by free water, such as cerebrospinal fluid (CSF), helping to differentiate between free and restricted water diffusion within brain tissue. During early life, the brain experiences significant changes, including neurite growth and branching. NODDI allows researchers to quantitatively assess these changes, providing valuable information on normal brain maturation and the effects of developmental disorders. NODDI can detect these microscopic changes, contributing to a better understanding of processes related to cognitive decline and age-related neurodegenerative diseases. By identifying early biomarkers for these conditions, NODDI can significantly aid in developing preventive and therapeutic methods.

Although NODDI offers detailed information on the microstructure of the brain, it has limitations, such as its inability to distinguish between different populations of fibers within a voxel, especially in the developing brain, where fiber tract maturation and myelination are crucial. The assumptions made when modeling the diffusion signal and the need for validation studies with preterm or newborn human tissue samples are also significant challenges. Despite correlations with histological changes in certain conditions, the clinical relevance of NODDI indices is not yet fully established. The slow clinical adoption of NODDI may be due to factors beyond the computational cost. To address these issues, there is a need for improvements in specificity, validation in preterm and neonatal populations, and optimization of acquisition protocols for clinical use. In addition, extensive longitudinal studies are required to understand the progression of neurodevelopmental changes and the impact of NODDI-detectable microstructural changes on cognitive and behavioral outcomes. Addressing these challenges could make NODDI a more powerful tool in neonatal neuroimaging and contribute to the early diagnosis and prognosis of neurological conditions in the developing brain.

2.4 Tractography

Diffusion MRI-based tractography is a sophisticated imaging method used to chart white matter tracts within the brain by following the diffusion of water molecules along neural fibers [23]. This technique provides comprehensive three-dimensional representations of brain connectivity, revealing the links among various brain regions, and has demonstrated its worth in both research and clinical environments, especially for studying brain development (**Figure 3**). Using dMRI, tractography depends on the directional properties of water diffusion in the brain, enabling it to determine the alignment of white matter fibers. Several tractography algorithms have been created to reconstruct white matter tracts, including deterministic tractography, probabilistic tractography, and global tractography, each offering distinct benefits and computational considerations.

Tractography has become a crucial tool for understanding brain development, providing valuable insights into the progression of brain connectivity from early childhood to adulthood. During brain development, white matter tracts undergo

DOI: http://dx.doi.org/10.5772/intechopen.1007630

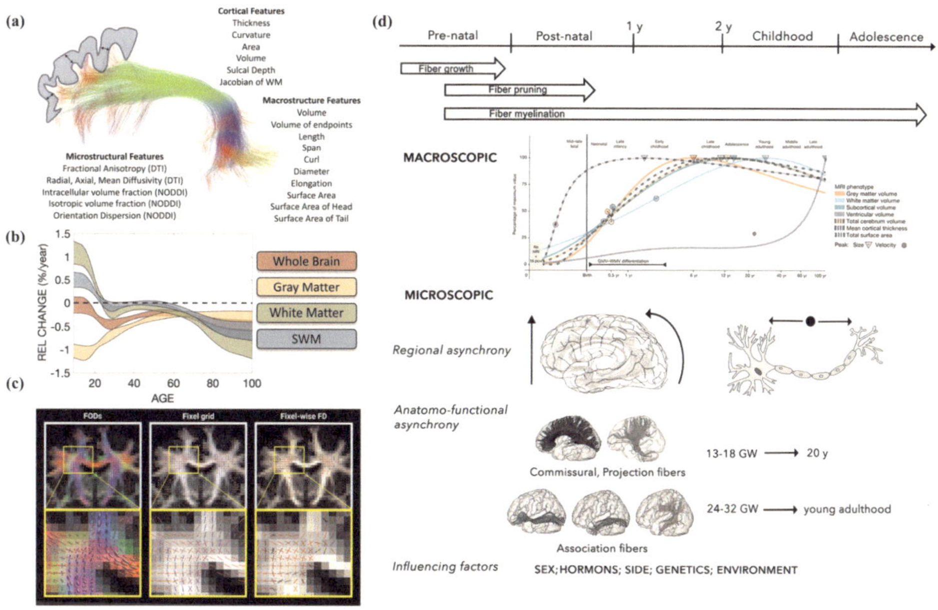

Figure 3.
(a) Microstructural, macrostructural, and cortical features associated with 63 white matter bundles (a) Adapted from: Ref. [24] (b) The relative volume change in percentage change per year for whole brain, gray matter, white matter, and subcortical white matter (SWM) tissue types. (b) Adapted from: Ref. [25]. (c) The derivation of a fixel "grid" and fixel-wise apparent fiber density, provides insight into the computation and visualization of apparent fiber density metrics (c) Adapted from: Ref. [26]. (d) A comprehensive summary of the critical properties of brain structural network development, highlighting the macroscopic and microstructural developmental trends and their associated characteristics (d) Adapted from: Ref. [27].

notable changes, including improvements in myelination, fiber density, and complexity, all of which can be observed and measured using tractography (**Figure 3**). Tractography has also been essential for studying neurodevelopmental conditions such as autism, attention deficit hyperactivity disorder (ADHD), and dyslexia. By comparing the white matter connectivity of affected individuals with normally developing controls, researchers can identify irregularities in neural pathways that may be at the root of cognitive and behavioral symptoms. In addition, tractography helps to explore how specific tracts contribute to cognitive functions such as language, memory, and executive function.

However, tractography faces challenges in accurately delineating and tracking white matter pathways, especially in regions of fiber crossing. Manual extraction of streamlines using regions of interest (ROIs) is considered the gold standard, but it is time-consuming and operator-dependent, leading to variability in results. Validation of tractography methods, especially in the developing brain, requires further research with larger, longitudinal, multisite, and multirace datasets. Future research should focus on improving the accuracy and precision of tractography in mapping complex fiber configurations in the developing brain, addressing data quality and acquisition variability, and validating methods in diverse populations. By addressing these limitations, tractography has the potential to provide new insight into brain structure and function in clinical and research settings.

dMRI has greatly advanced our understanding of the brain connectome through tractography-based structural connectivity. However, a primary limitation is the challenge of brain parcellation, which influences the topological characteristics of structural connectomes. The lack of consensus on the optimal parcellation approach and the need for a more precise description of parcellation methods hinder the reproducibility and comparability of the results. Current tractography techniques also need improvement in robustly tracking fibers within and between multiple gray matter regions to ensure reliable connectivity indicators. The translation of the findings of the group study into individual patients remains a significant gap and it is necessary to validate MRI markers derived from structural properties for personalized rehabilitation strategies and clinical settings. Future research may benefit from a shift toward graph-theory-based analysis to provide a more comprehensive characterization of structural connectivity.

2.5 Fixel-based analysis

Fixel-based analysis (FBA) represents an advanced technique that offers more detailed information on the fiber populations within each voxel [26]. This powerful method quantifies individual fiber populations within a single voxel, a departure from traditional methods that provide only averaged diffusion metrics per voxel (**Figure 4(c)**). FBA distinguishes and examines individual fiber bundles, known as "fixels," within each voxel, leading to a more precise depiction of brain microstructure, especially in regions with intricate fiber configurations. Quantitative metrics, such as fiber density (FD), fiber cross-section (FC), and fiber density and cross-section (FDC), are calculated for each fixel, providing detailed information on the microstructural integrity and morphology of individual fiber populations.

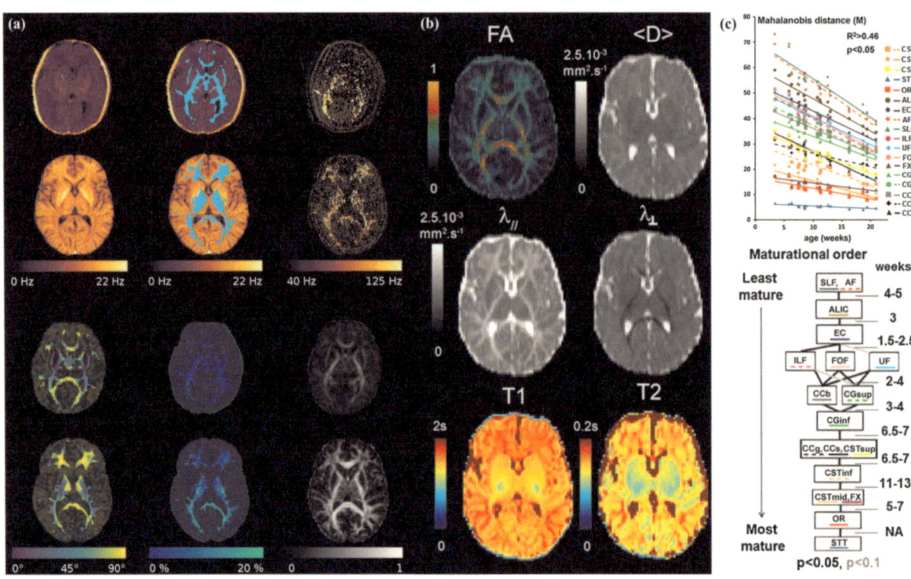

Figure 4.
(a) The parameter maps in axial view for a representative newborn and an adult subject. In the adult subject, elevated R2 in white matter compared to surrounding gray matter was observed, while this contrast was inverted in the newborn subject. (a) Adapted from: Ref. [28]. (b) Quantitative maps of magnetic resonance imaging (MRI) parameters for a 6-week-old infant were presented, and the bundle maturational order revealed by the Mahalanobis distance was discussed. (c) maturational relationships between the bundles were represented as a graph, with relative maturational delays between the bundles or bundle groups being indicated. (b-c) Adapted from: Ref. [29].

Group comparisons and statistical analyses are conducted on fixel metrics to detect variations and alterations in white matter tracts.

However, FBA faces challenges related to tractography quality, which is influenced by various factors such as the MRI scanner, protocol, and algorithms, leading to variability in results. The application of FBA in the developing brain is particularly challenging due to the dynamic nature of brain maturation, and current frameworks may not adequately capture changes in white matter microstructure during development. Addressing these limitations requires the development of advanced diffusion models, the integration of machine learning algorithms, and large-scale multisite studies to understand normative brain development patterns and identify biomarkers for developmental disorders.

3. Applications in the developing brain

3.1 Brain development

In early childhood, advanced dMRI techniques show that white matter in the brain improves quickly (**Figure 1**). This is because myelination, which helps signals travel between neurons, occurs rapidly at this time. It supports important developmental milestones such as motor skills and language acquisition. During adolescence, dMRI techniques reveal that the development of white matter tracts continues at a slower pace. This period is marked by the refinement of neural networks and synaptic pruning, which are crucial for the development of advanced cognitive functions such as abstract reasoning and impulse control. In adulthood, the maturation of white matter tracts stabilizes (**Figure 5**), and advanced dMRI techniques help identify age-related changes in white matter integrity.

Several studies have focused on the use of constrained spherical deconvolution (CSD) and FBA to study the development of white matter in preterm-born baby groups [30–33]. Studies have shown positive connections with age in FD, FC, and FDC in white matter during childhood and early childhood, indicating an active period of dynamic white matter maturation. Comprehensive investigations using data from the Human Connectome Project (dHCP) also show similar developmental trends of age-related nonlinear increases in FD between preterm and full-term babies [31]. Throughout infancy and early childhood, widespread nonlinear increases in NDI have been observed during the first 3 years of life [34], with continued increases until

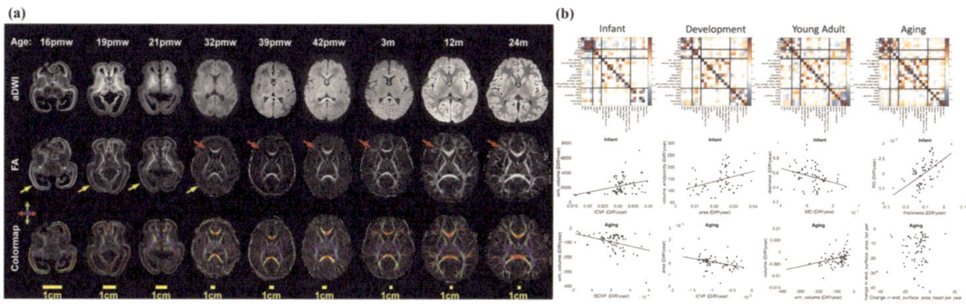

Figure 5.
(a) dMRI contrast in the fetal and infant brain spanning from 16 postmenstrual weeks (pmw) to 2 years (24 months) of age. (a) Adapted from: Ref. [5]. (b) The age associations of microstructure, macrostructure, and cortical features of pathways exhibit significant relationships. (b) Adapted from: Ref. [24].

7.5 years of age [32, 33], followed by a plateau in adolescence. These nonlinear increases in NDI observed primarily in white matter, are believed to reflect myelination and axonal packing and are significant features of white matter development during early life. Studies from childhood to adolescence indicate that NDI shows more pronounced age-related changes in gray matter and white matter compared to DTI measures [35]. Longitudinal findings also suggest age-related increases in NDI in children between the ages of 6 and 13 years [36]. Both NDI and ODI show rapid increases in early childhood that decelerated during adolescence. More longitudinal investigations are needed to better understand individual rates of change during the early stages of brain development and their correlation with behavioral development.

However, the biophysical interpretation of dMRI metrics is not always straightforward. For example, the meaning of NDI, ODI, and FD in the context of brain development is still a subject of debate, and these metrics can be influenced by a variety of factors, including axonal diameter, density, and myelination. Advanced diffusion MRI techniques are still limited in their ability to differentiate between different cell types and tissue microenvironments, such as the distinction between the contributions of axonal and glial cells to the signal. In addition, longitudinal dMRI studies are essential for understanding brain development but are logistically challenging and require careful tracking of the subject and data harmonization over time. Future research directions should focus on improving data acquisition, improving modeling techniques, integrating multimodal imaging, and translating these techniques into clinical practice to fully realize their potential. For example, applying machine learning algorithms to extract more meaningful information from dMRI data and to predict developmental outcomes or identify early markers of neurological conditions. In addition, we investigated how genetic and environmental factors interact to influence brain development using dMRI as a readout of brain microstructure.

3.2 Autism spectrum disorder (ASD)

ASD is a complex developmental disorder characterized by difficulties in social interaction and communication, repetitive behaviors, and narrow interests. The varied ways in which the condition presents in individuals make it challenging to identify specific brain indicators. However, there is consistent evidence pointing to disruptions in the connectivity of white matter in ASD. Advanced techniques in dMRI provide detailed information on the microstructural properties of white matter and the arrangement of neural connections, contributing to our understanding of the underlying neurobiology of ASD and offering potential biomarkers for early diagnosis and intervention.

Previous studies on diffusion microstructure have shown that ASD individuals exhibit different axonal anatomy compared to typically developing individuals, including structural variances in neuronal WM, with ASD associated with lower FA and higher diffusivity [37]. A study using NODDI discovered elevated extracellular water and reduced neurite density in individuals with ASD in key tractography bundles in the brain [38]. Another study used constrained spherical deconvolution to compare axonal volume differences between individuals with ASD and participants that typically develop using fixed-based analysis. The analysis revealed that participants with ASD had a significantly lower fiber density cross-section [37]. The disturbances in the development of white matter and connectivity observed in individuals with ASD may be the basis for certain core symptoms of the disorder.

The past few decades have seen an explosion of ASD research, yet a comprehensive understanding of the neurobiological underlying principles of the disorder remains elusive. This lack of clarity hinders the development of targeted therapeutic interventions. The vast array of studies has yielded a multitude of findings; however, many of these have not been replicated or have been called into question due to methodological flaws or inconsistencies. One of the critical limitations of dMRI in the context of ASD is its spatial and temporal resolution. Although the technique can capture the white matter tracts of the brain and provide insight into connectivity, it may not be sufficiently precise to visualize the synaptic or neuronal abnormalities that are hypothesized to be the basis for the core characteristics and heterogeneity of ASD. If resolution does not allow for the detection of these subtle abnormalities, dMRI may not be the optimal tool for parsing the nuances of ASD.

3.3 Attention deficit hyperactivity disorder (ADHD)

The dMRI has revealed alterations in the white matter tracts in individuals with ADHD, improving our understanding of the neural basis of the disorder. Studies investigating white matter abnormalities in ADHD using DTI have yielded diverse findings, with a lack of consensus among the research. A recent investigation has revealed a negative correlation between FA values in specific white matter tracts, the polygenic risk score for ADHD, and increased use of screen time [39]. Furthermore, a study using DKI found that individuals with isolated ADHD exhibited greater microstructural complexity in certain regions of the brain compared to controls that typically develop. A previous study using multishell dMRI with biophysical modeling identified a decrease in dendrite density and volume in certain white matter fiber tracts in the frontal lobe of the brain in patients with ADHD [40].

The early development stage represents both a critical period of neurodevelopment and a stage of significant vulnerability to unfavorable environmental conditions and adverse experiences that can influence childhood development. A recent study used NODDI to examine the effects of increased risk factors for adverse childhood experiences on brain development in children, with and without ADHD [41]. This research underscores the impact of early adverse childhood experiences on brain development in children with and without ADHD, demonstrating the sensitivity of NODDI to these neurodevelopmental disparities. This study may serve as a foundation for the development of targeted interventions for children at high risk for adverse childhood experiences.

Fortunately, the realm of neuroimaging and machine learning (ML) research has seen a surge in studies aimed at accurately classifying neurological disorders such as ADHD using various MRI modalities. However, there is significant variability in the methodologies, which can lead to overestimation of the performance of the model. Despite the progress reported, translating ADHD-related findings into clinical practice remains challenging due to inconsistencies in research findings, sample heterogeneity, and limited comprehensive assessment tools beyond MRI. The complexity and heterogeneity of ADHD call for a more nuanced approach, such as large-scale longitudinal studies, to capture the diverse nature of the disorder. Furthermore, the relationship between structural and functional networks in the context of ADHD requires further elucidation for a better understanding of the pathophysiology of the disorder.

3.4 Cerebral palsy

Cerebral palsy (CP) is the most common neuromotor disorder in children. It is the result of various nonprogressive brain injuries that occur at different stages of fetal or infant brain development, such as brain infections, periventricular leukomalacia, malformations, or perinatal strokes. Various disruptions in early brain development lead to varying sizes of lesions, directly affecting the integrity of gray and white matter in all regions of the brain and the central nervous system pathways [42].

Tractography has shed light on the role of white matter injury in the pathophysiology of CP and motor impairments. In children with CP, injury is often observed in the corticospinal tract (CST), posterior thalamic radiations (PTR), superior thalamic radiations (STR), and areas of the corpus callosum (CC) [43]. In the preterm infant brain, abnormal white matter is believed to be the result of a complex interaction between impaired axonal development and degeneration [44]. By quantifying micro and macrostructural changes in white matter, CSD-derived fixel-based metrics should be able to better capture abnormal white matter development after delays or initial direct injury to preoligodendrocytes or immature axons, with or without aberrant recovery in the pathogenesis of CP. Fixel-based white matter measures in the main sensorimotor tracts derived from CSD have been shown to be independently associated with the early diagnosis of cerebral palsy in very premature infants scanned at term equivalent age [30].

However, multicenter studies are necessary to uncover early indicators that can include a variety of impairments. Genetic studies have suggested that genetic factors may play an important role in the development of CP, leading to the potential identification of specific genes associated with the condition. Advanced imaging modalities, along with metabolic and genetic tests, play a vital role in revealing subtle changes in brain structure and function. This multidisciplinary approach can help to understand the complex interplay between genetic predispositions, metabolic processes, and brain development.

3.5 Genetic disorders

Offers insights into how genetic mutations impact brain development and the integrity of white matter. Although age-related changes in brain structure have been observed in white matter microstructure [45], most studies on imaging genetics are restricted to cross-sectional research designs, except studies on newborn twins [46]. A recent longitudinal study that investigated the age-related development of NODDI measures among singletons from infancy through early childhood found that age has a positive correlation with NDI, but little to no correlation with ODI [47]. Longitudinal twin imaging studies that span adolescence and adulthood could potentially provide a better understanding of age-related changes in genetic and environmental influences compared to dividing groups into younger and older age ranges in cross-sectional studies.

In a twin study using HARDI, Shen et al. [48] discovered that the white matter fiber modeled by the fiber orientation distribution (FOD) function is more heritable than FA. The fiber orientation distribution function may present a more precise depiction of axonal fiber organization and might be more sensitive to underlying genetic factors in regions with large populations of crossing fibers. For example, Kochunov et al. [49] indicated that regions closer to the thalamus (the center of the brain in the Montreal Neurological Institute space) showed a higher heritability of FA compared to distal regions. The qualitative observation that Falconer's heritability in FA decreases at the edge of white matter and cortical gray matter likely supports this previous finding. Furthermore, the preliminary voxel-based Falconer heritability estimates in the study largely validate the findings based on regions of interest (ROIs). Future investigations will conduct additive genetic, common environmental, and unique environmental (ACE) modeling at the voxel level and explore potential regional changes in heritability. Furthermore, twin modeling of NODDI measures can be expanded to cover the entire brain to examine the genetic foundation of microstructural features in cortical and subcortical gray matter. For example, orientation dispersion should capture the fanning and complexity of neurite fiber orientation [50], which are crucial attributes for brain development and neurodegenerative disorders.

Advanced dMRI techniques have shown promise in the study of genetic disorders by providing a detailed view of the brain's microstructure. However, while large-scale morphometric measurements are valuable, they do not offer detailed information on the brain's microstructure, which is crucial for understanding genetic disorders. Secondly, the interpretation of the dMRI findings can be subjective, leading to variability in the results. Objective interpretation and standardized assessment methods are necessary. Advanced dMRI measures could monitor the impacts of lifestyle factors on health and contribute to personalized treatments, but their applicability to a broad spectrum of functions and symptoms must be carefully considered.

3.6 Preterm infants

Infants born preterm have a particular vulnerability to disrupting early neurodevelopmental processes, placing them at high risk of motor, cognitive, and behavioral deficits that become more evident later in childhood [51]. Preterm birth is also associated with an increase in the risk of psychiatric disorders in adulthood [52]. Studies have shown that DKI-derived measurements have revealed differential cortical microstructural profiles and maturational patterns in the cortex, emphasizing the improved ability of DKI to measure rapidly changing microstructural features of neurodevelopment [5]. Preterm infants scanned at term equivalent age have been found to have reduced fractional anisotropy, fiber density, and fiber cross-section in various white matter regions [53]. Higher fixel measurements were associated with improved neurodevelopmental outcomes at 1 year in preterm infants of term equivalent age. Furthermore, higher fixel measurements were associated with better math computation ability in children, regardless of their gestational age at birth [54]. In contrast, very prematurely born children exhibited lower fixel measurements in the main white matter tracts [55].

Researchers have studied the development of the brain in preterm infants compared to those born at full term [56]. They found that preterm infants showed a delay in brain maturation compared to term infants. In addition to the white matter of the brain, researchers are also studying the microstructure of gray matter [57]. They have observed changes in gray matter microstructure in premature infants, indicating a developmental interplay between gray and white matter growth. Furthermore, a recent study reported widespread decreases in gray matter microstructure in preterm newborns compared to term-born infants [58]. Researchers have used NODDI to study the effects of very preterm birth on the development of white matter in children aged 5, 6, and 7 years [55, 59, 60]. They found that children born very preterm had lower NDI [55], which was associated with lower intelligence quotient (IQ) and worse semantic performance. The researchers also found that differences in the microstructure of white matter were associated with cognitive outcomes and processing speed in both groups of children [59, 60]. This research highlights the need for further study into the biological mechanisms supporting differential neurodevelopmental and cognitive outcomes in children born very prematurely and with very low birth weight.

Advanced dMRI techniques offer valuable insight into the brain microstructure of preterm infants, but they face certain limitations when applied to this vulnerable population. The constraints of scan time and stability of sedation in neonatal patients must be carefully considered when designing imaging protocols. Furthermore, the unique microstructural environment of preterm infants requires caution in interpreting advanced dMRI measures, as the norms for these metrics may not directly apply. Genetic factors and methodological choices also influence the accuracy and applicability of advanced dMRI in this context. Developing optimized protocols for quantitative MRI analysis tailored to the specific needs of preterm infants is crucial to monitor disease progression and response to treatment.

3.7 Hypoxic: Ischemic encephalopathy (HIE)

dMRI is useful for assessing the severity of brain damage in newborns with HIE, which is vital for predicting outcomes and planning treatment. At 6 months of age, dMRI indicated a possible decrease in brain network function and organization as neuromotor deficits increased after neonatal encephalopathy. DTI and functional MRI, using a passive motor task at 40 to 48 weeks postconceptional age after perinatal brain injury, revealed that FA and functional connectivity of the right supplemental motor area can predict cerebral palsy at 2 years of age. The neonatal brain injury pattern of the Neonatal Research Network was identified as a reliable indicator of neurodevelopmental outcomes between 6 and 7 years of age. Furthermore, a recent extensive study revealed that infants who showed better neurodevelopmental results at 1 and 2 years of follow-up showed higher FD, FC, and FDC in the corticospinal tract, midbrain, and corpus callosum. This suggests improved information transfer capability due to a larger number of neurons, improved myelination, thicker nerve bundles, and various combinations. Another recent study on infants with HIE reported a decrease in FD in widespread white matter tracts in infants with HIE compared to controls [61].

Advanced dMRI has shown great potential to study brain microstructure in the context of hypoxic-ischemic encephalopathy (HIE), a condition that often affects newborns. However, there are several limitations to consider when applying this technique to HIE. The dynamic nature of cerebrospinal fluid can affect the precision of apparent diffusion coefficient (ADC) values, making it challenging to predict brain injury and its chronic effects. Outcome measures for early evaluation of treatment effects and long-term prognostication are crucial, and advanced dMRI techniques such as NODDI show promise in providing more in-depth information.

4. Discussion

4.1 General challenges

dMRI is a valuable tool to explore the microstructure of the brain. However, conducting neuroimaging in neonates, infants, and pediatric populations presents several unique challenges. Advanced diffusion imaging acquisitions, such as HARDI or multishell protocols, require longer scan times and present significant difficulties in obtaining motion-free data.

Participant motion substantially affects the dMRI data, leading to blurring, ghosting, dropout, and other artifacts that degrade image quality, especially in people who have difficulty remaining still during scanning, such as infants and young children. In addition to motion, loud acoustic sounds, and long scan times, the small size of the brain in newborns and young children can also pose challenges in obtaining an adequate signal-to-noise ratio (SNR) and requires increased resolution to avoid effects of partial volume artifacts, consequently increasing scan times [62]. Furthermore, signal inhomogeneities and variability in tissue characteristics are observed in the early stages of development due to asynchronous temporal development of myelination across brain regions. The underdeveloped infant brain, characterized by a high water content and low myelin, is accompanied by differential diffusion characteristics, including longer relaxation times differential diffusivity patterns, and signal inhomogeneities [63] compared to adults. These challenges lead to poor gray-white matter contrast and can complicate brain segmentation methods [64].

In the context of the developing brain, advanced dMRI techniques, such as DTI, DKI, and NODDI, can provide valuable information about myelination, axonal diameter, and tissue microstructure. These metrics can be used as biomarkers to predict developmental outcomes and monitor the effects of interventions. However, translating these findings into clinical practice requires further validation. Studies are needed to correlate diffusion magnetic resonance metrics with clinical outcomes and establish normative values for different age groups and developmental stages. In addition, there is a need for automated and reliable post-processing tools that can handle the complexity of diffusion data and provide actionable insights to clinicians.

Another of the main limitations of dMRI in clinical settings is the variability in image quality due to differences in the hardware, software, and acquisition parameters of the MRI scanner. To ensure consistent and reliable results, it is essential to standardize these factors between different centers. Multicenter collaborations, such as those involved in the Human Connectome Project and the Alzheimer's Disease Neuroimaging Initiative, have demonstrated the feasibility of collecting and sharing diffusion data with strict protocol adherence, which can help mitigate scanner-related biases.

4.2 Future directions

4.2.1 Spherical mean technique

The spherical mean technique (SMT) is an advanced approach used in dMRI that provides unique advantages for the analysis and interpretation of diffusion data [65], especially in the context of the developing brain. By focusing on the mean signal over all gradient directions for a given diffusion weighting (b value), this technique simplifies the analysis of diffusion data. This averaging process eliminates the effects of anisotropy, allowing the extraction of microstructural parameters that are independent of fiber orientation. The resulting isotropic component provides valuable insight into tissue characteristics, such as cell density and membrane permeability. Biophysical models are used to calculate microstructural parameters, including intra- and extracellular volume fractions, diffusivities, and axonal diameter, from the spherical mean signal. SMT is particularly well suited for studying complex processes such as myelination, axonal growth, and synaptic pruning in the developing brain due to its ability to provide orientation-independent microstructural information.

However, SMT requires assumptions and oversimplifications regarding neural tissue characteristics, which impacts the interpretation of derived metrics, especially in disease states. Its accuracy and precision, particularly in complex tissue structures, have yet to be fully evaluated. SMT may also produce discrepancies in metrics compared to traditional diffusion-weighted imaging, attributed to imposed constraints. Future research should focus on refining the technique and validating its metrics in the context of the developing brain, addressing inherent assumptions, and developing new methodologies to better resolve complex fiber configurations. In addition, new diffusion encoding strategies hold promise in capturing microstructural features of tissues under healthy and pathological conditions, potentially aiding in clinical translation.

4.2.2 Soma and neurite density imaging (SANDI)

SANDI, or Soma and Neurite Density Imaging, is a sophisticated dMRI method created to distinguish and measure soma (cell body) and neurite (axons and dendrites) densities [66]. It is especially useful for studying the developing brain, where complex and dynamic changes occur during growth and maturation. SANDI goes beyond traditional diffusion models by incorporating multicompartment biophysical models that individually define the diffusion of water within the soma and neurite compartments. This distinction allows for accurate quantification of cellular and neurite densities, providing a comprehensive view of tissue microstructure. Due to significant structural changes in the developing brain, such as the growth and maturation of neurons and glial cells, as well as the establishment and refinement of neural connections, SANDI is well suited to investigate these processes.

SANDI shows promise in characterizing white and gray matter in the brain. However, one challenge is to minimize acquisition time while maintaining image quality, particularly in areas susceptible to distortion. The precision and precision of SANDI in complex tissue structures, such as those in the developing brain, need further evaluation. The potential of SANDI for clinical translation is also a significant consideration for future research. Although SANDI offers promise for noninvasive imaging of soma and neurite density, it requires further refinement and validation, particularly in the context of the developing brain.

4.2.3 Time-dependent diffusion MRI

Time-dependent diffusion MRI (td-dMRI) is a sophisticated imaging technique that provides deep insights into the dynamic characteristics of tissue microstructure [67, 68], especially in the investigation of the developing brain. Conventional dMRI methods assess the diffusion of water molecules over a fixed diffusion time, offering limited details about tissue microstructure dynamics (**Figure 2(e)**). In contrast, td-dMRI involves collecting diffusion measurements over multiple diffusion times, generating a comprehensive data set that reveals temporal alterations in water diffusion (**Figure 6**). This approach uses variations in diffusion time during image acquisition to monitor changes in diffusion signal over time and obtain information regarding the dimensions and permeability of the tissue microstructure. The acquired data generate quantitative parameters that describe the temporal progression of diffusion, providing insights into microstructural characteristics such as cell size, packing density, and membrane permeability. Furthermore, td-dMRI can be used to track the development of brain tissues over time, highlighting modifications in cell size, density, and myelination advancement (**Figure 1**). However, td-dMRI faces challenges such as long acquisition times and complex data analysis, limiting its widespread adoption in clinical and research settings. Future research aims to refine the time-dependent

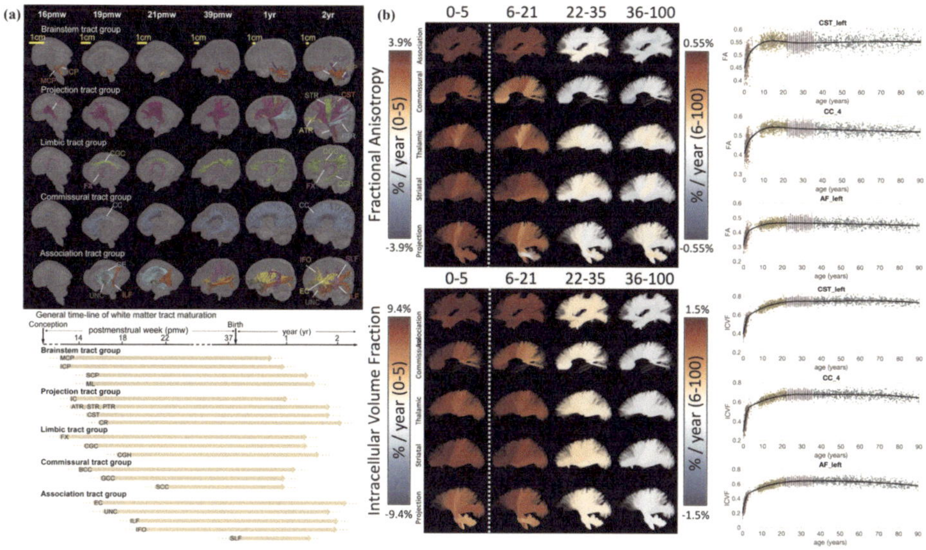

Figure 6.
(a) The development of white matter tracts in the fetal and infant brain from 16 postmenstrual weeks to 2 years. The study categorized various types of tracts and established a comprehensive timeline for white matter maturation across different tracts and tract groups. (a) Adapted from: Ref. [5]. (b) Distinct lifespan trajectories of white matter microstructure. Trajectories of fractional anisotropy (FA) and intracellular volume fraction (ICVF) were displayed in color, representing the percentage difference per year for each cohort in a cross-sectional manner, with data points plotted against age for three selected pathways. (b) Adapted from: Ref. [24].

diffusion (TDD) methodologies for clinical viability, integrate TDD with other MRI modalities for a comprehensive assessment of brain tissue microstructure, and deepen understanding of the biophysical basis of the metrics of TDD.

5. Conclusions

Advancements in dMRI technologies and techniques over the past two decades have paved the way for significant progress in our understanding of brain maturation in health and disease. The studies discussed suggest the remarkable potential for advanced and multishell dMRI in describing the cellular architecture of early brain maturation and detecting structural abnormalities in various disorders of central pathophysiology. Advanced dMRI is a rapidly evolving field with significant potential to improve our understanding of the developing brain. With a deeper understanding of the developmental patterns that occur in early brain development detected by advanced and biophysical models of dMRI comes novel opportunities for the early detection, diagnosis, and treatment of conditions during the early stages of the establishment of neural foundations.

Acknowledgements

This work was supported by the National Key R&D Program of China (Nos. 2023YFE0118600 and 2023YFF1204800). This work was supported by the National

Natural Science Foundation of China (Nos. 62201265, 62371107, 62101365, 62172228, 61971214) and the Guangdong Province Natural Science Foundation of Guangdong Province of China (No. 2023A1515012093).

Conflict of interest

The authors declare that they have no conflict of interest.

Author details

Ye Wu[1*], Lanxiang He[1], Xinyuan Zhang[2] and Fan Zhang[3]

1 Nanjing University of Science and Technology, Nanjing, China

2 Southern Medical University, Guangzhou, China

3 University of Electronic Science and Technology of China, Chengdu, China

*Address all correspondence to: wuye@njust.edu.cn

References

[1] Basser PJ, Pierpaoli C. Microstructural and physiological features of tissues elucidated by quantitative-diffusion-tensor MRI. Journal of Magnetic Resonance. 1996;**111**(3):209-219

[2] Uhl Q et al. Quantifying human gray matter microstructure using neurite exchange imaging (NEXI) and 300 mT/m gradients. Imaging Neuroscience. 2024;**2**:1-19

[3] Somerville LH et al. The lifespan human connectome project in development: A large-scale study of brain connectivity development in 5–21 year olds. NeuroImage. 2018;**183**:456-468

[4] Park B-Y et al. Connectome-wide structure-function coupling models implicate polysynaptic alterations in autism. NeuroImage. 2024;**285**:120481

[5] Ouyang M et al. Delineation of early brain development from fetuses to infants with diffusion MRI and beyond. NeuroImage. 2019;**185**:836-850

[6] Makropoulos A et al. Regional growth and atlasing of the developing human brain. NeuroImage. 2016;**125**:456-478

[7] Dean DC III et al. Modeling healthy male white matter and myelin development: 3 through 60 months of age. NeuroImage. 2014;**84**:742-752

[8] Batalle D et al. Annual research review: Not just a small adult brain: Understanding later neurodevelopment through imaging the neonatal brain. Journal of Child Psychology and Psychiatry. 2018;**59**(4):350-371

[9] Bystron I et al. Development of the human cerebral cortex: Boulder committee revisited. Nature Reviews Neuroscience. 2008;**9**(2):110-122

[10] Tau GZ, Peterson BS. Normal development of brain circuits. Neuropsychopharmacology. 2010;**35**(1):147-168

[11] Luby JL. Handbook of Preschool Mental Health: Development, Disorders, and Treatment. New York, NY: Guilford Press; 2009

[12] Gilmore JH et al. Imaging structural and functional brain development in early childhood. Nature Reviews Neuroscience. 2018;**19**(3):123-137

[13] Altimus CM et al. The next 50 years of neuroscience. Journal of Neuroscience. 2020;**40**(1):101-106

[14] Mori S, Zhang J. Principles of diffusion tensor imaging and its applications to basic neuroscience research. Neuron. 2006;**51**(5):527-539

[15] O'Donnell LJ, Westin C-F. An introduction to diffusion tensor image analysis. Neurosurgery Clinics of North America. 2011;**22**(2):185-196

[16] Descoteaux M. High angular resolution diffusion MRI: From local estimation to segmentation and tractography [thesis]. France: Université Nice Sophia Antipolis; 2008

[17] Lu H et al. Three-dimensional characterization of non-Gaussian water diffusion in humans using diffusion kurtosis imaging. NMR in Biomedicine. 2006;**19**(2):236-247

[18] Martinez-Heras E et al. Diffusion-weighted imaging: Recent advances and applications. Seminars in Ultrasound, CT and MRI. 2021;**42**(5):490-506

[19] Zhang H et al. Axon diameter mapping in the presence of orientation dispersion with diffusion MRI. NeuroImage. 2011;**56**(3):1301-1315

[20] Alexander DC et al. Imaging brain microstructure with diffusion MRI: Practicality and applications. NMR in Biomedicine. 2019;**32**(4):e3841

[21] Zhang F et al. MK-curve improves sensitivity to identify white matter alterations in clinical high risk for psychosis. NeuroImage. 2021;**226**:117564

[22] Zhang H et al. NODDI: Practical in vivo neurite orientation dispersion and density imaging of the human brain. NeuroImage. 2012;**61**(4):1000-1016

[23] Yamada K et al. MR Tractography: A review of its clinical applications. Magnetic Resonance in Medical Sciences. 2009;**8**(4):165-174

[24] Schilling KG et al. White matter tract microstructure, macrostructure, and associated cortical gray matter morphology across the lifespan. Imaging Neuroscience. 2023;**1**:1-24

[25] Schilling KG et al. Superficial white matter across development, young adulthood, and aging: Volume, thickness, and relationship with cortical features. Brain Structure and Function. 2023;**228**(3–4):1019-1031

[26] Dhollander T et al. Fixel-based analysis of diffusion MRI: Methods, applications, challenges and opportunities. NeuroImage. 2021;**241**: 118417

[27] De Benedictis A et al. Structural networking of the developing brain: From maturation to neurosurgical implications. Frontiers in Neuroanatomy. 2023;**17**. DOI: 10.3389/fnana.2023.1242757

[28] Bartels LM et al. Orientation dependence of R2 relaxation in the newborn brain. NeuroImage. 2022;**264**: 119702

[29] Kulikova S et al. Multi-parametric evaluation of the white matter maturation. Brain Structure and Function. 2015;**220**(6):3657-3672

[30] Chandwani R et al. Early micro- and macrostructure of sensorimotor tracts and development of cerebral palsy in high risk infants. Human Brain Mapping. 2021;**42**(14):4708-4721

[31] Liu T et al. Diffusion MRI of the infant brain reveals unique asymmetry patterns during the first-half-year of development. NeuroImage. 2021;**242**: 118465

[32] Dimond D et al. Early childhood development of white matter fiber density and morphology. NeuroImage. 2020;**210**:116552

[33] Dimond D et al. Maturation and interhemispheric asymmetry in neurite density and orientation dispersion in early childhood. NeuroImage. 2020;**221**: 117168

[34] Fenchel D et al. Development of microstructural and morphological cortical profiles in the neonatal brain. In: Cerebral Cortex. Vol. 30(11). New York, N.Y.: Oxford University Press; 1991, 2020. pp. 5767-5779

[35] Mah A et al. Detailing neuroanatomical development in late childhood and early adolescence using NODDI. PLoS One. 2017;**12**(8):e0182340

[36] Geeraert BL et al. A multiparametric analysis of white matter maturation during late childhood and adolescence. Human Brain Mapping. 2019;**40**(15): 4345-4356

[37] Dimond D et al. Reduced white matter fiber density in autism spectrum disorder. In: Cerebral Cortex. Vol. 29(4). New York, N.Y.: Oxford University Press; 1991, 2019. pp. 1778-1788

[38] Andica C et al. Neurite orientation dispersion and density imaging reveals white matter microstructural alterations in adults with autism. Molecular Autism. 2021;**12**(1):48

[39] Yang A et al. Longer screen time utilization is associated with the polygenic risk for attention-deficit/hyperactivity disorder with mediation by brain white matter microstructure. eBioMedicine. Jun 2022;**80**:104039. DOI: 10.1016/j.ebiom.2022.104039. Epub 2022 May 1

[40] Wu D et al. Developmental score of the infant brain: Characterizing diffusion MRI in term- and preterm-born infants. Brain Structure and Function. 2020; **225**(8):2431-2445

[41] Hare MM et al. Adverse childhood experiences predict neurite density differences in young children with and without attention deficit hyperactivity disorder. Developmental Psychobiology. 2022;**64**(1):e22234

[42] Mailleux L et al. The relationship between neuroimaging and motor outcome in children with cerebral palsy: A systematic review-part B diffusion imaging and tractography. Research in Developmental Disabilities. 2020;**97**: 103569

[43] Parikh NA et al. Early detection of cerebral palsy using sensorimotor tract biomarkers in very preterm infants. Pediatric Neurology. 2019;**98**:53-60

[44] Volpe JJ. The encephalopathy of prematurity–brain injury and impaired brain development inextricably intertwined. Seminars in Pediatric Neurology. 2009;**16**(4):167-178

[45] Lebel C, Beaulieu C. Longitudinal development of human brain wiring continues from childhood into adulthood. Journal of Neuroscience. 2011;**31**(30):10937-10947

[46] Lee SJ et al. Quantitative tract-based white matter heritability in 1- and 2-year-old twins. Human Brain Mapping. 2019;**40**(4):1164-1173

[47] Lynch KM et al. Magnitude and timing of major white matter tract maturation from infancy through adolescence with NODDI. NeuroImage. 2020;**212**:116672

[48] Shen KK et al. Investigating brain connectivity heritability in a twin study using diffusion imaging data. NeuroImage. 2014;**100**:628-641

[49] Kochunov P et al. Heritability of fractional anisotropy in human white matter: A comparison of human connectome project and ENIGMA-DTI data. NeuroImage. 1 May 2015;**111**: 300-311

[50] Fukutomi H et al. Neurite imaging reveals microstructural variations in human cerebral cortical gray matter. NeuroImage. 15 Nov 2018;**182**:488-499

[51] Saigal S, Doyle LW. An overview of mortality and sequelae of preterm birth from infancy to adulthood. Lancet (London, England). 2008;**371**(9608): 261-269

[52] Nosarti C et al. Preterm birth and psychiatric disorders in young adult life. Archives of General Psychiatry. Jun 2012;**69**(6):610-617

[53] Shi J et al. Initial application of diffusional kurtosis imaging in

evaluating brain development of healthy preterm infants. PLoS One. 2016;**11**(4): e0154146

[54] Pannek K et al. Fixel-based analysis reveals alterations is brain microstructure and macrostructure of preterm-born infants at term equivalent age. NeuroImage. Clinical. 2018;**18**:51-59

[55] Kelly CE et al. Long-term development of white matter fibre density and morphology up to 13 years after preterm birth: A fixel-based analysis. NeuroImage. 2020;**220**:117068

[56] Galdi P et al. Neonatal morphometric similarity networks predict atypical brain development associated with preterm birth. In: Wu G et al., editors. Connectomics in NeuroImaging. Cham: Springer International Publishing; 2018. pp. 47-57

[57] Eaton-Rosen Z et al. Longitudinal measurement of the developing grey matter in preterm subjects using multi-modal MRI. NeuroImage. 2015;**111**: 580-589

[58] Kimpton JA et al. Diffusion magnetic resonance imaging assessment of regional white matter maturation in preterm neonates. Neuroradiology. 2021; **63**(4):573-583

[59] Sato J et al. Early nutrition and white matter microstructure in children born very low birth weight. Brain Communications. 2021;**3**(2):fcab066

[60] Sato J et al. White matter alterations and cognitive outcomes in children born very low birth weight. NeuroImage. Clinical. 2021;**32**:102843

[61] Jeong J-W et al. Neonatal encephalopathy prediction of poor outcome with diffusion-weighted imaging connectome and fixel-based analysis. Pediatric Research. 2022;**91**(6): 1505-1515

[62] Afacan O et al. Evaluation of motion and its effect on brain magnetic resonance image quality in children. Pediatric Radiology. 2016;**46**(12): 1728-1735

[63] Dubois J et al. MRI of the neonatal brain: A review of methodological challenges and neuroscientific advances. Journal of Magnetic Resonance Imaging. 2021;**53**(5):1318-1343

[64] Wang L et al. LINKS: Learning-based multi-source IntegratioN frameworK for segmentation of infant brain images. NeuroImage. 2015;**108**: 160-172

[65] Henriques RN et al. Microscopic anisotropy misestimation in spherical-mean single diffusion encoding MRI. Magnetic Resonance in Medicine. 2019; **81**(5):3245-3261

[66] Palombo M et al. SANDI: A compartment-based model for non-invasive apparent soma and neurite imaging by diffusion MRI. NeuroImage. 2020;**215**:116835

[67] Bogusz F et al. Diffusion-relaxation scattered MR signal representation in a multi-parametric sequence. Magnetic Resonance Imaging. 2022;**91**:52-61

[68] Wu Y et al. Relaxation-diffusion spectrum imaging for probing tissue microarchitecture. In: Greenspan H et al., editors. Medical Image Computing and Computer Assisted Intervention – MICCAI 2023. Vol. 14227. Cham: Springer Nature Switzerland; 2023. pp. 152-162

Section 2

Functional Imaging and Clinical Diagnostics

Chapter 2

Connection between Diseases and Neuroimaging of the Nervous System

Tse Jung Liu

Abstract

Neuroimaging refers to techniques that can directly or indirectly image the functional, structural, and pharmacological properties of the nervous system. In clinical diagnosis, physicians can first infer the location of nerve damage based on clinical symptoms, then confirm the clinical symptoms based on imaging examination results, and further clarify the cause and disease of the patient. As neuroimaging has gradually become widely used in medical institutions around the world, neuroimaging technology has now reached a diversified level and is applied to disease/injury identification in different fields based on its different principles. However, there is currently no neuroimaging technology that can accurately identify specific neurological diseases alone. Most neurological diseases have obvious symptoms and corresponding neuroimaging features in the early stages. This chapter summarizes the neuroimaging features and their possible corresponding diseases and proposes a correlation diagram between symptoms, neuroimaging features, and neurological diseases. It is expected to improve the accuracy and convenience of clinical physicians in applying neuroimaging technology.

Keywords: neuroimaging, nervous system, clinical diagnosis, disease identification, injury identification

1. Introduction

Neuroimaging encompasses a variety of techniques used to create visual representations of brain structure and function. The main goals of neuroimaging are to help diagnose brain disorders, assess the severity of conditions, and monitor changes over time [1]. There are many types of neuroimaging technologies, each with different imaging principles and detection purposes. The most commonly used techniques include magnetic resonance imaging (MRI), functional magnetic resonance imaging (fMRI), computed tomography (CT), and positron emission tomography (PET). MRI is a non-invasive imaging technique that uses powerful magnets to create a strong magnetic field, forcing protons in the patient's body to align with that field. The faster the protons in a patient's body rearrange themselves, the brighter the images produced by the MRI [2]. MRI has been widely used as a biomarker for Alzheimer's disease (AD) [3–5]. Functional MRI is a type of MRI scan that can show activity in specific areas of the brain.

IntechOpen

It is special in that it can track blood flow to different parts of the brain. The areas of the brain that work the hardest appear brighter on the X-ray scan [6]. fMRI can also be used to detect neurological diseases of the brain, including AD and degenerative dementia [6–9]. A computerized tomography scan is often called a CT scan. A CT scan uses a combination of X-rays and computer technology to create images of the inside of the body. It can be performed with contrast agents, allowing for a clearer view of the specific organ or tissue being studied [10]. CT can be used to identify a variety of abnormalities associated with cerebrovascular disease, including hemorrhage, ischemia, edema, meningitis, and infarction [11]. PET is an imaging test that helps reveal the metabolic, or biochemical, function of tissues and organs. PET scans use a radioactive drug called a tracer to show typical and atypical metabolic activity. PET scans can often detect abnormal metabolism of the tracer in the vein before they become apparent on other imaging tests. The tracer is then collected in areas of the body with more metabolic or biochemical activity, further pinpointing the location of the disease. PET imaging is often combined with CT or MRI, referred to as PET-CT or PET-MRI scans [12]. PET can effectively detect neurodegenerative diseases (NDs), including AD and dementia [13–15]. For the reasons stated above, different types of neuroimaging techniques produce different neuroimaging results and interpretation methods. Therefore, how to help clinicians quickly and accurately use neuroimaging to assist in the diagnosis of patients' diseases is the focus of this chapter. This chapter will present the neuroimaging characteristics corresponding to various neurological diseases, hoping to improve the convenience and accuracy of subsequent neuroimaging interpretation by clinicians.

2. Central nervous system

The central nervous system (CNS) consists of the brain and spinal cord. It is part of the nervous system. The other part is the peripheral nervous system, which consists of nerves that connect the brain and spinal cord to the rest of the body. The brain is protected by the cranial cavity, and the spinal cord begins behind the brain, runs along the center of the spine, and ends in the lower back at the waist. The brain and spinal cord are enclosed in three protective membranes called the meninges. The retina, optic nerve, olfactory nerve, and olfactory epithelium are sometimes considered part of the CNS along with the brain and spinal cord. This is because they connect directly to brain tissue without interfering with nerve fibers [16].

The nervous system is made up of basic units called neurons. Neurons are also called brain cells. Neurons are arranged in networks that carry electrical and chemical messages between the brain and the rest of the body. The brain is composed of gray matter (GM) and white matter (WM), of which GM consists of nerve cell bodies and blood vessels. WM is made up of axons (long cords extending from nerve cells). They are surrounded by myelin, a fatty substance that insulates the axon and helps electrical messages travel faster along the axon [17].

2.1 The brain

The brain is the most complex organ in the human body. The cerebral cortex contains an estimated 15 billion to 33 billion neurons, each of which is connected to thousands of other neurons. The brain is the central control module of the human body, coordinating various activities. It is responsible for functions ranging from body movement to hormone production, memory production and emotional perception.

The brain consists of different parts such as the cerebrum, cerebellum, thalamus, hypothalamus, and brainstem, of which the cerebrum is the largest part of the brain. It controls intelligence, memory, personality, emotions, speech, sensation, and motor abilities [17]. The cerebrum is divided into two hemispheres, the left and right, connected by a band of nerve fibers in the center of the brain called the corpus callosum. The cerebrum is roughly divided into four lobes. The main functions of each lobe are shown in **Table 1**.

Deep in the brain are the thalamus and hypothalamus. The thalamus carries messages to and from the lobes and controls movement and memory. The hypothalamus controls appetite, thirst, and body temperature. It also produces hormones that control the release of other hormones from the pituitary gland [17].

The basis of the brain is the brainstem. It is important for breathing, blood pressure, and the body's response to danger. **Table 2** describes some specific brain regions in more detail.

2.2 Spinal cord

The spinal cord is a string of nerve tissue that extends from the brainstem to the center of the spine and nearly the entire back. It carries messages between the brain and body as well as performing other tasks. It is made up of millions of nerve cells that send messages in the form of electrical nerve signals between the brain and the rest of the body. Starting from the brainstem, there are 31 spinal nerves that enter the spinal cord. Along its length, it connects with the nerves of the peripheral nervous system (PNS) that extend from the skin, muscles, and joints. The spinal cord also controls downward reflex movements of the neck. Circuits within the spine can also produce more complex movements [17].

2.3 WM and GM

The CNS can be roughly divided into WM and GM. In general, the brain consists of the outer cortex of the GM and the inner regions of the WM. Both types of tissue contain glial cells, which protect and support neurons. WM is mainly composed of axons and oligodendrocytes, while GM is mainly composed of neurons. Changes in GM and WM have long been considered to be associated with cognitive and neurological diseases [1]. Michel et al. [18] used regularized structural equation models to predict cognitive performance measured by GM and WM and found that the amount of GM and WM differed in different cognitive performances. Different indicators

Lobes	Main functions
Temporal lobe	Important for processing sensory input and giving it emotional meaning. It is also involved in the formation of long-term memory and some aspects of speech perception.
Occipital lobe	The visual processing area of the brain includes the visual cortex.
Parietal lobe	The parietal lobe integrates sensory information, including language processing, touch, spatial awareness, and navigation.
Frontal lobe	The frontal lobe is located in the front of the brain and contains most of the dopamine-sensitive neurons involved in attention, reward, short-term memory, motivation, and planning.

Table 1.
Main functions of each cerebral lobe.

Brain region	Main functions
Basal ganglia	Involved in the control of voluntary movements, procedural learning, and decisions about which motor activities to perform. Diseases that affect this area include Parkinson's disease (PD) and Huntington's disease (HD).
Cerebellum	Mainly involved in precise motor control, but also in language and attention. If the cerebellum is damaged, the main symptom is impaired motor control, called ataxia.
Broca district	This small area on the left side of the brain is important for language processing. When impaired, a person will find it difficult to speak but can still understand language. Stuttering is sometimes associated with inactivity in Broca's area.
Corpus callosum	A wide band of nerve fibers connecting the left and right hemispheres. It is the largest WM structure in the brain and allows the two hemispheres to communicate. Dyslexic children have smaller corpus callosum; left-handers, ambidextrous people, and musicians often have larger ones.
Medulla oblongata	It extends below the skull and is involved in involuntary functions such as vomiting, breathing, sneezing, and maintaining correct blood pressure.
Hypothalamus	The hypothalamus, about the size of an almond, is located above the brainstem and secretes a variety of neurohormones that influence body temperature control, thirst, and hunger.
Thalamus	The thalamus, located in the center of the brain, receives sensory and motor input and forward it to the rest of the cerebral cortex. It is involved in the regulation of consciousness, sleep, awareness, and alertness.
Amygdala	There are two amygdalae deep in the temporal lobe. They are involved in decision-making, memory, and emotional responses, especially negative emotions.

Table 2.
Specific brain regions responsible for function.

within had different predictive abilities, and the regions/areas that best predicted cognitive performance varied between indicators.

2.4 Central glial cells

Glial cells, also known as glial cells, are often referred to as the support cells of neurons. In the brain, they outnumber nerve cells 10 to 1. In the Panax notoginseng nervous system, each cell has a different type of system. The types and functions of glial cells in the CNS are shown in **Table 3**.

Glial cells in the CNS and PNS are thought to be involved in the pathogenesis of NDs. In diseases, especially NDs glial cells can exhibit progressive dysfunction and damage neurons [19]. Wang et al. [20] reviewed the relationship between glial cells and neurological diseases. Pattern recognition receptors (PRRs) such as Toll-like receptors (TLRs) and NOD-like receptors mediate microglia-associated neuroinflammation in PD. Mitochondria are important organelles that play a role in neuronal degeneration and glial cell activation. Aging and Alzheimer's disease promote the expression of inflammatory genes in the hippocampus, suggesting that inflammatory responses are enhanced in aging and Alzheimer's disease. By analyzing spatiotemporal specific co-expression networks in AD, microglial and astrocyte genes were more enriched than neuronal genes, further suggesting that glial cells are involved in AD. In addition, communication between glial cells and neurons plays an important role in regulating signal transduction and immune responses in the CNS

Types of glial cells	Main functions
Stellate cells	These cells have many processes and anchor the neuron to its blood supply. They also regulate the local environment by removing excess ions and recycling neurotransmitters.
Oligodendrocytes	Responsible for forming myelin—the thin layer that covers nerve cells, allowing them to send signals quickly and efficiently.
Ependymal cells	Lines the spinal cord and ventricles (fluid-filled spaces) of the brain. They produce and secrete cerebrospinal fluid (CSF) and use whip-like cilia to maintain cerebrospinal fluid circulation.
Radial glial cells	Serves as a scaffold for new nerve cells during the formation of the embryonic nervous system.

Table 3.
Types of glial cells in the central nervous system.

and PNS. Under pathological conditions, microglia and astrocytes release pro-inflammatory factors, which affect the phagocytic function of glial cells and damage neurons, aggravating neuroinflammation. In addition to the production of inflammatory factors by glial cells, communication between glial cells and neurons can also be mediated by extracellular vesicles (EVs).

The cranial nerves are made up of 12 pairs of nerves that emerge directly from the brain through holes in the skull rather than traveling along the spinal cord. These nerves collect and send messages between the neck and head. Of these 12 pairs of nerves, the olfactory and optic nerves originate from the forebrain and are considered part of the CNS, where the olfactory nerve transmits information about smells from the upper part of the nasal cavity to the olfactory area located at the base of the brain. Optic nerves carry visual information from the retina to the brain's primary visual

Diseases	Main functions
Vascular disease	Vascular disease affects blood flow within the nervous system, often leading to a lack of oxygen to the brain, which can lead to tissue death in the affected areas [21].
Trauma	Depending on the location of the injury, symptoms can vary widely, ranging from paralysis to mood disorders [22].
Degenerate	It involves the gradual degeneration of dopamine-producing cells in the nucleus basalis. In some cases, PD may occur in the spinal cord or brain, others include multiple sclerosis, AD, etc. [23].
Tumor	Tumors can damage the nervous system and cause a range of symptoms, depending on where they develop [24].
Infect	Some microorganisms and viruses can invade the central nervous system during infection [25].
Structural defects	Structural defects, such as birth defects.
Autoimmune diseases	The immune system produces antibodies that mistakenly attack the body's own cells [26].

Table 4.
Central nervous system diseases.

nuclei, and each optic nerve is composed of approximately 1.7 million nerve fibers [16].

There are many diseases that affect the CNS. These conditions can be divided into different categories, summarized in **Table 4**.

3. Basic interpretation methods of neuroimaging and neuroimaging characteristics caused by physical injury

The previous section briefly introduced the human nervous system and related diseases. The focus of this section is how to clarify clinical symptoms and make further diagnoses based on imaging manifestations. Therefore, correct interpretation of neuroimaging is essential for clinicians to make a diagnosis. First, before interpreting neuroimaging, the orientation of the images must be determined. CT and MRI are currently the most commonly used brain neuroimaging techniques in countries around the world [1]. **Table 5** summarizes the characteristics of different brain tissues on neuroimaging, including GM, WM, cerebrospinal fluid (CSF) or water, fat, air, bone, or calcification and edema.

Figure 1 shows the neurological images from CT and MRI. According to the judgment principles in **Table 5**, we suggest that two or more different neuroimaging

Tissue	T1 – Weighted	T2 – Weighted	X-Ray
GM	Gray	Light gray	Shades of gray
WM	White	Dark gray	Shades of gray
CSF or water	Black	White	Shades of gray
Fat	White	Black	Shades of gray
Air	Black	Black	Black
Bone or Calcification	Black	Black	White
Edema	Gray	White	Shades of gray

Table 5.
Appearance of Commonly Scanned Tissues [27].

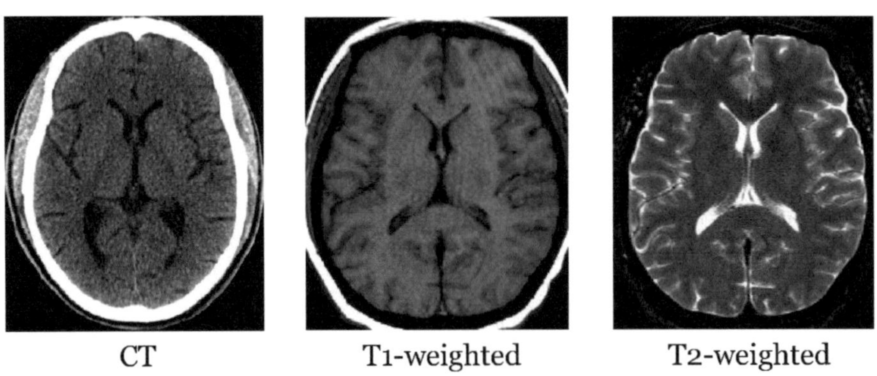

Figure 1.
(a) The location of the "hand tubercle" area. (b) The location of the paracentral lobule.

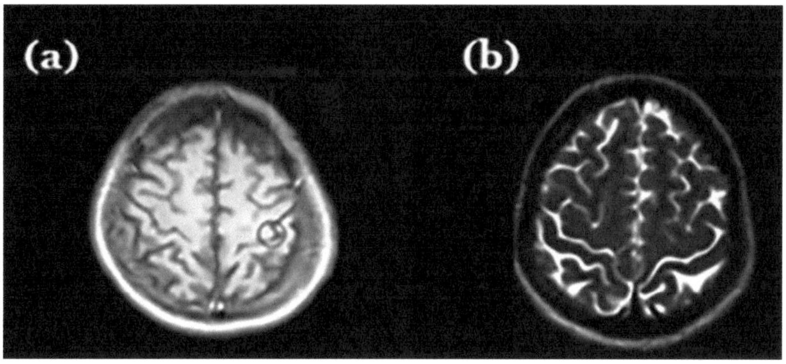

Figure 2.
Differences between CT and MRI neuroimaging.

techniques can be used to identify tissues and symptoms in the images. We can also see from **Figure 2** that T1-weighted scans show better anatomical details than T2-weighted scans and T2-weighted scans can show pathological abnormalities, including fluid abnormalities.

The cerebral cortex is divided into 52 areas (Brodmann area). Each brain region is just a core area that performs a certain function. Other parts of the cortex have similar functions. When a certain area of the brain is damaged, other related brain areas may have a certain compensatory effect [28].

The structure of the brain can be roughly divided into the telencephalon, midbrain, brainstem, cerebellum, and ventricular system. The following subsections outline the characteristic locations of neuroimaging effects of regional injuries in various parts of the brain, which can provide clinicians with diagnostic convenience.

3.1 Neuroimaging characteristics of damage or lesions in frontal lobe regions

The frontal lobe can be roughly divided into the cortical motor area, premotor area, cortical lateral visual center, writing center, motor language center, frontal lobe, defecation and urination center, and other areas. Each area of the brain is responsible for different functions [16].

The motor areas of the human cerebral cortex are located in the precentral gyrus and paracentral lobule. The motor areas are characterized by crossing and reversal. Contralateral movement disorders occur after injury. Minor injuries to this area can cause contralateral unilateral hemiplegia, while severe injuries can cause flaccid paralysis or spastic paralysis [22, 28]. Lesions in the lower motor area will result in contralateral tongue paralysis [22, 28, 29]. Injury to the upper motor area may result in paralysis of the corresponding area of the contralateral limb. Damage to the paracentral lobule can lead to contralateral lower limb paralysis and difficulty urinating and defecating [22]. Combined injuries may result in paralysis on the other side of the body [22]. The "hand tubercle" area of the precentral gyrus is primarily responsible for controlling the muscles of the contralateral hand.

The frontal fusion zone includes areas 9 to 12 of the frontal lobe. Specific structures include the orbital gyrus, medial surface of the frontal lobe, superior frontal gyrus, middle frontal gyrus, and anterior part of the inferior frontal gyrus. Nerve damage in this area can lead to abnormal mental status and cognition, which may be accompanied by hypoactivity and urinary incontinence, decreased orbital gyrus stimulation ability, frontal lobe ataxia, and intellectual decline. Inflammatory lesions can lead to autonomic nervous system dysfunction, such as respiratory and blood pressure disorders [29].

When the motor language center (Broca's area, located at the back of the inferior frontal gyrus) is damaged, people can understand what others say, but the speech is unclear and cannot be repeated. The middle frontal gyrus is also called the writing center. Its obvious characteristics are poor hand coordination and inability to write [22, 28].

If there is a large area of damage or lesions in the premotor area, it will cause fine motor disorders. It will also cause impaired ability to use the distal part of the contralateral limbs after the injury, which will manifest as frontal lobe ataxia after the injury. It is also associated with myotonia. After an injury, muscle tone increases, but muscle strength may be normal. Also related to the inhibition of primitive reflexes. After injury, primitive reflexes may occur on either the ipsilateral or contralateral side. It is related to the function of autonomic nerves, and autonomic nervous system dysfunction occurs after injury [22, 28].

The cortical motor area that controls contralateral lower limb movements and urination and defecation functions is located in the medial frontal lobe. After injury, movement disorders may occur primarily in the contralateral lower limb. The frontal association area is also distributed in the medial frontal lobe, and corresponding symptoms may appear after lesions.

In addition, damage to the basal surface of the frontal lobe may also involve the frontal pole, orbital surface of the frontal lobe, hypothalamus, olfactory nerve, and optic nerve, leading to intellectual, emotional, and recent memory impairments, as well as symptoms such as violent crying, panic, and palpitations [22].

3.2 Neuroimaging features of damage or lesions to parietal regions

The parietal lobe can be roughly further subdivided into three regions: the first somatosensory area (postcentral gyrus) the superior, and inferior parietal areas. The location of the first somatosensory area includes the postcentral gyrus and the posterior part of the paracentral lobule. It is responsible for sensation in the opposite half of the body. When irritating lesions appear, epilepsy will occur at the corresponding site on the contralateral side [22]. If destructive lesions occur, epilepsy can occur, [22] sensory impairment occurs. The location of the superior parietal area includes the superior parietal lobule, paracentral lobule, and precuneus. When diseased or injured, the sense of direction and movement is impaired [28]. The inferior parietal zone is located in the inferior parietal lobule and includes the supramarginal gyrus in front and the angular gyrus in the back. When lesions or injuries occur, dyslexia and dysgraphia can occur [6]. Guzman syndrome can occur due to lesions in the dominant angular gyrus, and lesions near the non-dominant angular gyrus may cause body image interference and structural application [28].

3.3 Neuroimaging characteristics of injuries or lesions in the temporal, occipital, and insular regions

The temporal lobe can be divided into auditory and non-auditory areas. The auditory area includes a first auditory area and a second auditory area. Non-auditory areas include speech formation areas, olfactory centers, and temporal lobe structures related to psychological and cognitive functions, and other areas. The functionality of each detailed area is described in the following sections.

3.3.1 Function of temporal lobe

The first auditory area is located in the middle of the transverse temporal gyrus and the middle of the superior temporal gyrus. Hearing impairment occurs after injury. Therefore, deafness will not occur after damage to the auditory center on one side but only after hearing loss, inability to locate the sound source, or auditory hallucinations [16, 22, 28].

The second listening zone is the auditory contact zone, which understands complex sounds and speech. The posterior part of the contact zone is Wernicke's area, which is responsible for language understanding. Wernicke's aphasia occurs after injury and is characterized by fluent language but an inability to understand what others are saying, poor comprehension, and low retelling ability [16, 22]. The non-auditory area includes the front end of the superior temporal gyrus, the middle temporal gyrus, the lateral surface of the inferior temporal gyrus, and the medial surface of the occipitotemporal gyrus. Damage to the language formation area (located in the posterior area 37 of the dominant middle temporal gyrus) can cause naming aphasia, which is characterized by the ability to understand other people's speech but often the inability to name objects [22].

After the olfactory center (located in the parahippocampal gyrus and hippocampal gyrus) is damaged, hallucinations, taste, and smell may be damaged or disappear [16]. The temporal lobe is related to mental and cognitive functions, and the anterior temporal lobe is related to memory, association, mental and visceral activities; the anterior temporal lobe is related to memory, association, mental and visceral activities, etc.; The hippocampus and amygdala in the anterior and medial temporal lobe have the function of regulating visceral activity and generating emotions. The nucleus is related to recent memory; the middle temporal gyrus, occipitotemporal gyrus, and amygdala are related to psychological cognitive functions. Memory loss, intellectual disability, mental and emotional abnormalities may occur after injury [22]. The lower half of the optic radiation in the visual conduction area is conducted through the temporal lobe to the lingual gyrus of the occipital lobe. This lesion results in blindness in the upper quarter of the contralateral visual field [22]. After the auditory reflex head-eye rotation area (located in area 22 of the lower part of the superior temporal gyrus) is injured, the eyes will squint to the opposite side [16, 22]. Dizziness and balance disorders may occur after damage to the vestibular center (the specific location is unknown, but it may be located in area 22) [22].

3.3.2 Function of occipital lobe

The occipital lobe can be further subdivided into the first visual area and the visual contact area according to their functions.

The first visual area (area 17, also known as the striatum area) is located on the medial surface of the occipital lobe, including the calcarine fissure, cuneate gyrus, and lingual gyrus. Receives visual fibers from the retina. Loss of visual field occurs after injury [22]. The visual contact area (including the second and third visual areas, namely areas 18 and 19) is the visual recognition area. After injury, visual hallucinations occur, and objects cannot be recognized [22, 28].

3.3.3 Function of insula

The function of the insula is very complex and related to emotion, pain, addiction, self-control, language function, autonomic nervous function, etc. It is currently impossible to subdivide the function of the insula [16].

3.4 Neuroimaging characteristics of injuries or lesions of the basal node, internal capsule, and corpus callosum

The basal ganglia include the caudate nucleus, lentiform nucleus (putamen, globus pallidus), claustrum, and amygdala. The broad basal ganglia also include the red nucleus, substantia nigra, and subthalamic nucleus. The caudate nucleus is mainly involved in motor regulation functions and is also related to cognitive functions. Lesions result in contralateral choreikinesia (chorea-like hypotonia and increased movement manifested by involuntary, irregular, faster movements), or non-pyramidal hemimotor syndrome. The main manifestations are inflexible movement, spontaneous movement accompanied by reduced movement, hemiplegia, etc. [16, 17, 22]. It can also manifest as basal ganglia aphasia, speech impairment, mild naming impairment, relative memory rehearsal, mood disorders, reduced emotional reactivity, apathy, depression, and memory loss [16, 17]. After the globus pallidus in the lentiform nucleus is damaged, tremors, increased muscle tone, bradykinesia, and hypokinesia will occur. Putamen damage is similar to caudate nucleus damage, but cognitive function decline generally does not occur [16, 17]. The internal capsule has a large number of nerve conduction fibers passing through it.

The anterior limb of the internal capsule contains the prethalamic radiation and the frontopontine tract, which are also involved in the regulation of movement. It is also involved in coordinating the movement of the throat muscles. Dysarthria may occur after the lesion. Lesions in the forelimb of the internal capsule on one side can cause ataxia in the contralateral limb, and lesions on both sides can cause mood disorders, involuntary crying, and involuntary laughter [16, 17].

The genu of the internal capsule contains cortical and nuclear tracts. Unilateral internal capsule lesions can cause contralateral central facial nerve palsy and tongue paralysis. Bilateral lesions cause bilateral nerve palsy and pseudobulbar palsy [16, 17].

The posterior limb of the internal capsule contains corticonuclear tracts, corticospinal tracts, thalamocortical fibers, auditory radiations, and visual radiations. "Three-hemisphere syndrome" (hemiplegia, hemianopia, and semi-sensory impairment) occurs after the lesion.

The corpus callosum is a complex fiber bundle connecting the left and right cerebral hemispheres. It is the connection and integration channel for the motor centers on both sides, the motor language center, the audio-visual center on both sides, and the emotional-cognitive functional areas.

Most activities require the integration of both cerebral hemispheres. When the corpus callosum is damaged, the function of the corresponding area is isolated. Therefore, the clinical manifestations after callosal lesions are very diverse. The main symptoms are mental disorders, such as inattention, memory loss, intellectual disability, personality changes, etc., and parietal lobes, fibers passing through the trunk of the corpus callosum connect the left and right posterior frontal lobes and parietal lobes, and the splenium of the corpus callosum mainly connects the left and right lobes. Lesions in the temporal and occipital lobes may cause functional impairments in the corresponding areas, and the affected functions may include vision, hearing, taste, smell, and language comprehension [22].

When the lesion occurs in the anterior 1/3 of the corpus callosum, (1) left-sided apraxia will occur. (2) Abnormal gait, muscle weakness, and speech impairment (the front part of the corpus callosum mainly connects the movement and motor speech centers). (3) Cognitive dysfunction and mental disorder. (4) Alien hand syndrome: It manifests as involuntary, uncontrollable, and purposeless movement of one upper limb or hand, accompanied by the patient's unfamiliarity and anthropomorphism of the affected limb. It mostly occurs on one side. Limb disease is caused by lesions of the non-dominant angular gyrus; alien hand syndrome is often characterized by an inability to control involuntary movements of the affected limb, resulting in hostility toward the affected limb. When the lesion occurs in 1/3 of the corpus callosum, related symptoms such as pseudobulbar palsy, ataxia, and mental confusion will occur. If the lesion occurs in the posterior 1/3 of the corpus callosum, related symptoms such as hemianopia, hearing impairment, and mental disorders will occur [16, 17].

Because physical injuries or lesions are acute, it is easier for clinicians to identify the location of the injury through neuroimaging and then speculate on possible symptoms or sequelae. Regarding what is mentioned in this section, neuroimages corresponding to the location of trauma in the body were compiled. The feature locations are shown in **Table 6** and **Figures 1, 3–15.**

Illness/ Disease	Cause	Symptoms	neuroimaging features/damage area	Corresponding neuroimaging
Physical trauma	Traumatic brain injuries caused by accidents/ irritating lesions/ lesions	Contralateral paralysis.	Motor cortex, precentral gyrus.	**Figure 1**
		Abnormal mental status, cognitive impairment, urinary incontinence.	frontal lobe	**Figure 3**
		Unable to repeat.	Broca's area	**Figure 4**
		unable to write	Middle frontal gyrus	**Figure 5**
		Fine motor impairment.	Premotor cortex	**Figure 6**
		Recent memory impairment, violent crying and laughing, and disturbance of consciousness.	Basal surface of frontal lobe	**Figure 7**
		Epilepsy, sensory impairment.	Postcentral gyrus, Posterior paracentral lobule	**Figure 8**
		Impaired sense of direction and movement	Superior Parietal Lobule, aracentral lobule, Precuneus	**Figure 7**
		Dyslexia and dysgraphia.	Inferior parietal lobule, Supramarginal gyrus, Angular gyrus.	**Figures 8–10**
		Hearing impairment.	Middle Transverse temporal gyrus, middle Superior temporal gyrus.	**Figure 11**

Illness/ Disease	Cause	Symptoms	neuroimaging features/damage area	Corresponding neuroimaging
		Wernicke's aphasia.	Wernicke's area	—
		Naming aphasia	Middle temporal gyrus.	**Figure 11**
		loss of taste, smell, and hallucinations.	Parahippocampal gyrus, Hippocampus.	**Figure 12**
		Amnesia, mental retardation.	Temporal Lobe	**Figure 11**
		Blindness in the upper 1/4 quadrant of the contralateral visual field.	Lower part of Gratiolet's bundle.	**Figure 13**
		Both eyes will squint to the opposite side.	Lower part of Superior temporal gyrus.	**Figure 11**
		Dizziness and balance disorders.	Vestibular system.	—
		Loss of vision.	Calcarine fissure, Fusiform gyrus, Lingual gyrus.	**Figure 14**
		Inability to recognize objects.	Visual contact area brain.	**Figure 15**
		Hemiplegia, basal ganglia aphasia.	Caudate nucleus, putamen.	—
		Increased muscle tone and decreased motor function.	Globus pallidus.	—
		Dysarthria.	Anterior limb of internal capsule.	—
		Contralateral central facial nerve palsy.	Genu of internal capsule.	—
		Hemiplegia, hemianopsia, hemisensory disorder.	Posterior limb of internal capsule.	—
		Ataxia, hemianopia, hearing impairment.	Corpus callosum.	—

Table 6.
Symptoms caused by physical trauma and their corresponding neuroimaging locations.

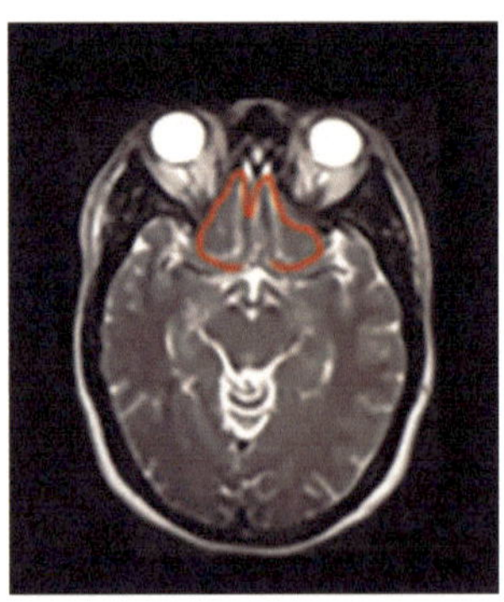

Figure 3.
Location of the frontal joint.

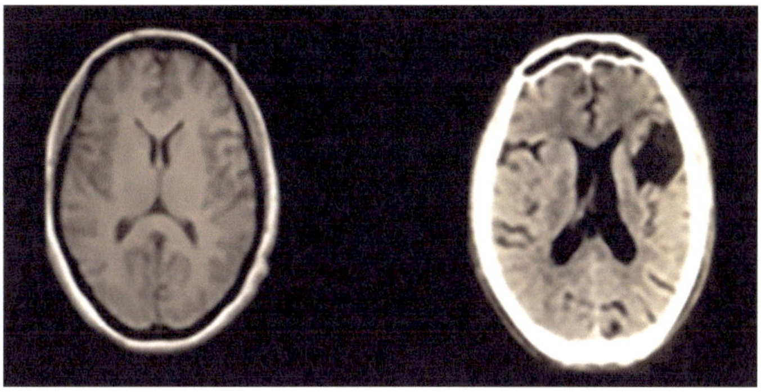

Figure 4.
Comparison of CT images between BROCA area lesions and normal subjects.

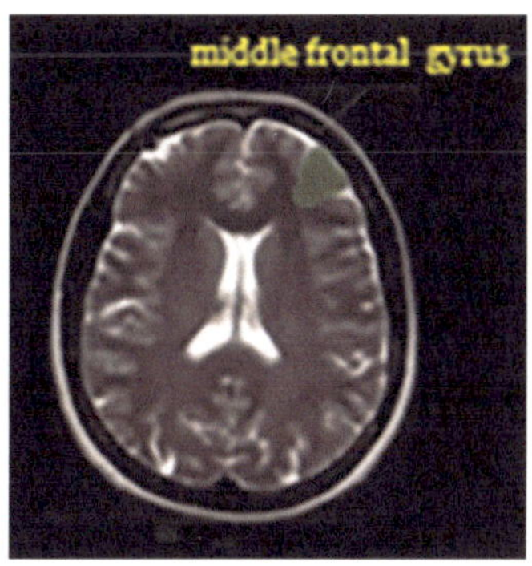

Figure 5.
Middle frontal gyrus location.

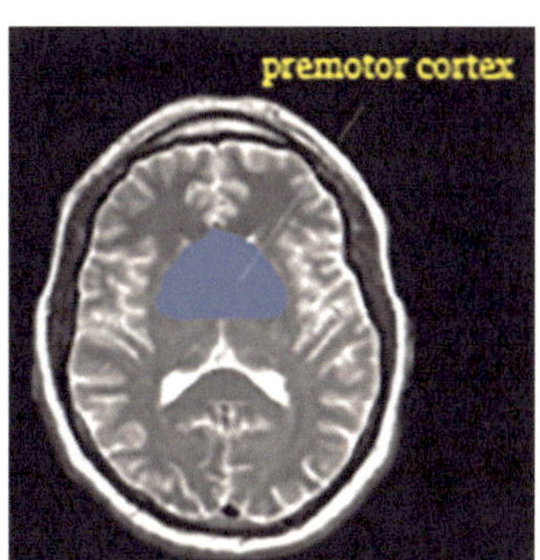

Figure 6.
The location of premotor cortex.

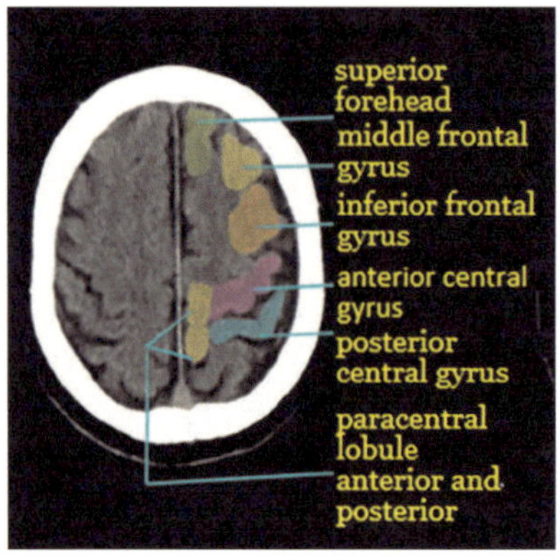

Figure 7.
Position of paracentral lobule.

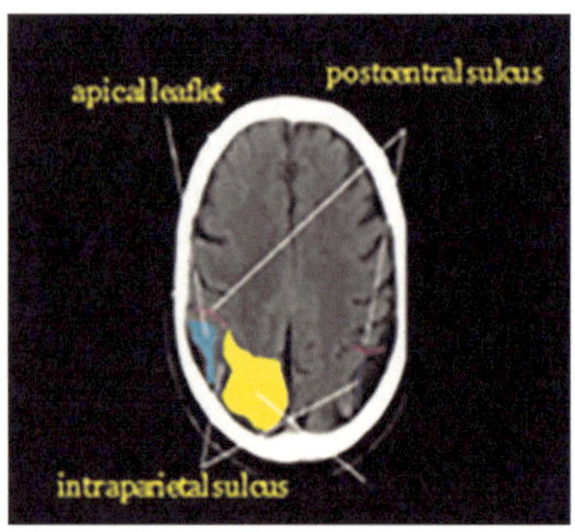

Figure 8.
Location of inferior parietal lobule.

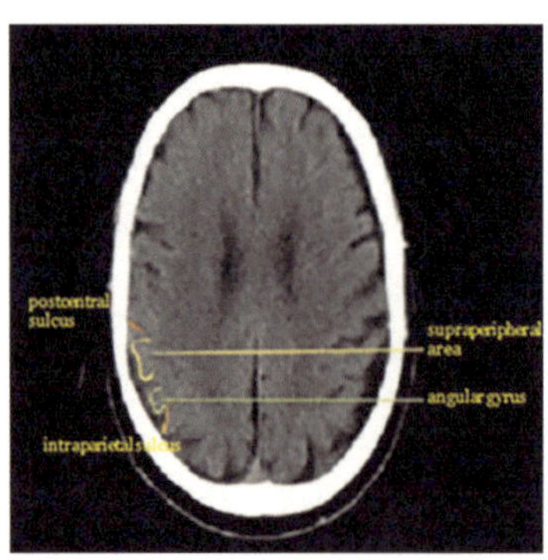

Figure 9.
The location of the angular gyrus.

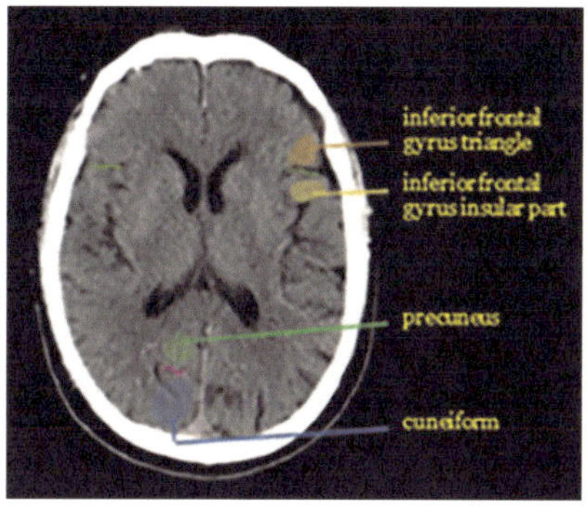

Figure 10.
Location of precuneus and cuneus.

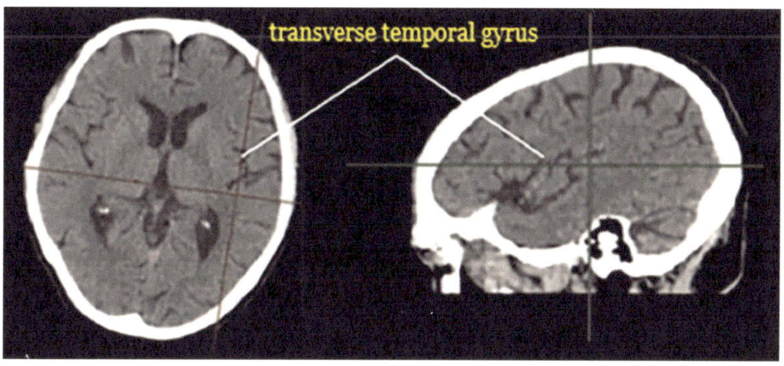

Figure 11.
Location of transverse temporal gyrus.

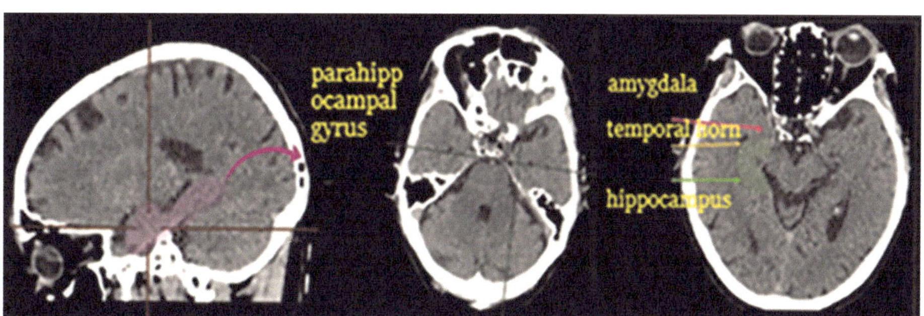

Figure 12.
The location of the parahippocampal gyrus.

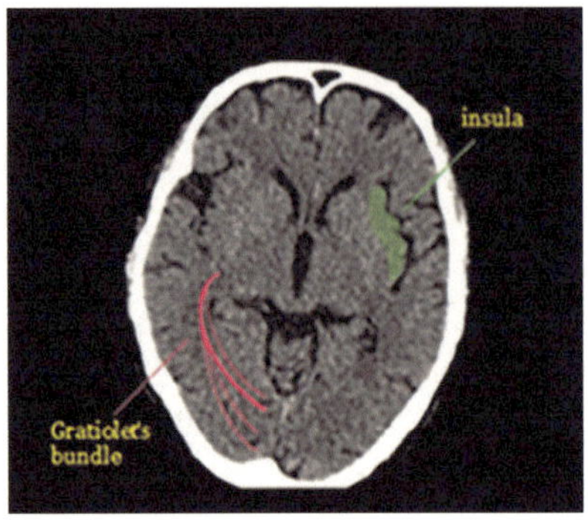

Figure 13.
Location of insula.

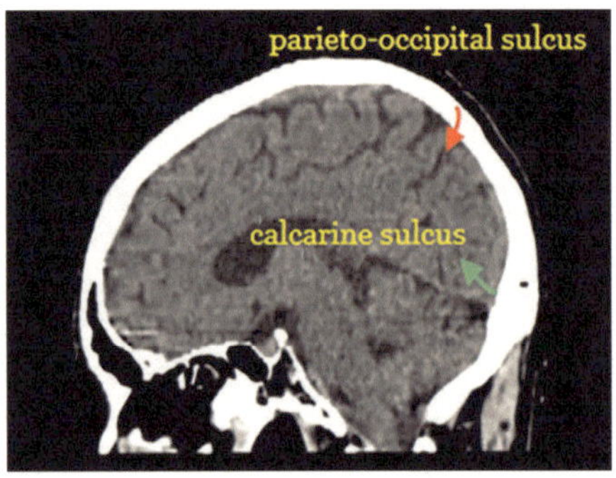

Figure 14.
Location of parieto-occipital sulcus and calcarine sulcus.

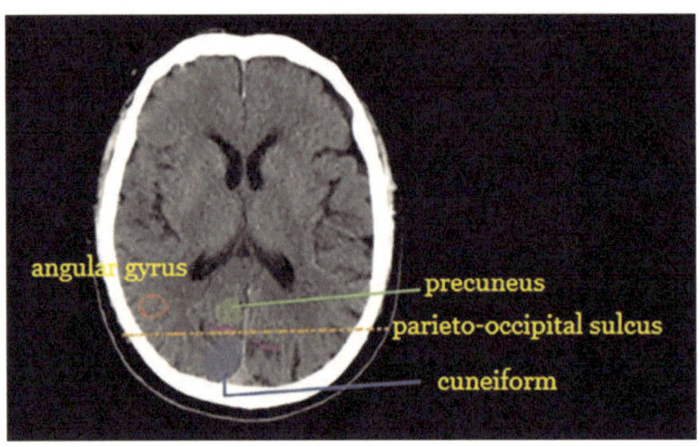

Figure 15.
Judgment of angular gyrus position.

4. Neuroimaging characteristics of specific neurological diseases

The previous section explained the impact of damage to various parts of the brain and nervous system on human functions. However, there are few reviews on auxiliary diagnosis and accelerated diagnosis of some common and special chronic neurological diseases. Chronic neurological diseases often eventually lead to dementia and can be divided into several types depending on the cause. In order to facilitate clinical physicians in diagnosing neurological diseases, this section comprehensively integrates the neuroimaging characteristics corresponding to common neurological diseases, improves the level of neurology, and facilitates physicians' clinical diagnosis.

4.1 Alzheimer's disease (AD)

AD is characterized by the abnormal accumulation of β-amyloid and tau proteins, forming neuritic plaques and neurofibrillary tangles (NFTs), respectively. These changes lead to neuronal dysfunction and death, followed by atrophy of selectively vulnerable brain networks and the emergence of clinical features, such as cognitive impairment. Current AD diagnostic criteria incorporate neuroimaging as a biomarker. There are markers of potential AD pathology in humans (amyloid PET scans) [15, 30–32].

Although the earliest site of AD pathology is often the accumulation of phosphorylation in the nuclei of brain stem cells, the earliest atrophy detected by MRI is in the brain. In the classic amnestic AD syndrome, atrophy of the hippocampus and precuneus occurs early [2–4, 15, 30].

Many patients with LOAD atrophy also often present with severe posterior involvement, whether or not they are symptomatic; this pattern often helps clinicians differentiate AD from other disorders that may present with a similar clinical syndrome. For example, corticobasal syndrome (CBS) is a disorder on the frontotemporal dementia (FTD) spectrum and may be associated with AD or frontotemporal lobar degeneration (FTLD) pathology. Patients with CBS due to underlying AD show pathology that is primarily parietal lobe atrophy, whereas patients with CBS due to FTLD pathology show pathology that is primarily frontal lobe atrophy [33]. Therefore, the finding of posterior atrophy (i.e., precuneus and posterior cingulate gyrus) on imaging studies suggests the presence of underlying AD pathology, as it is often a feature of the AD syndrome [33]. Atrophy in AD is not always symmetrical; for example, in patients with language-depleted variant primary progressive aphasia (lvPPA), in which AD is the underlying pathology, atrophy is first observed in the left temporoparietal junction. Viewing structural (T1) brain images in different planes often helps identify these anatomical features.

In AD diagnosis, functional imaging is often used as a supplement to structural imaging. Clinical practice has focused primarily on 18F-fluorodeoxyglucose [FDG]-PET and single-photon emission computed tomography (SPECT), but fMRI and even magnetoencephalography have elucidated unique associations with pathological and cognitive syndromes. Several studies have shown [15, 30–33] that the spatial pattern of hypometabolism in FDG-PET and the spatial pattern of hypoperfusion in SPECT overlap with the pattern of atrophy in MRI, especially in the inferior parietal cortex, lateral temporal cortex, posterior cingulate cortex, posterior temporal cortex, gyrus and/or precuneus.

4.2 Parkinson's disease (PD) and dementia with Lewy bodies (DLB)

PD and DLB are the most common NDs in the elderly. Pathologically, DLB and PD are characterized by the presence of intraneuronal α-synuclein "Lewy body" inclusions within neurons of the cortex, brainstem, and substantia nigra. The main distinguishing feature between PD and DLB is the timeline of symptom onset: DLB is diagnosed when cognitive symptoms precede or develop within the same year as motor symptoms, whereas DLB is diagnosed when motor symptoms precede cognitive decline by at least 1 year. When it appears at one year, DLB is diagnosed. When is PD diagnosed? The core feature of DLB is progressive cognitive decline in executive function, visuospatial function, and memory, which usually appears in the late stages of the disease [34, 35].

Brain MRI in patients with DLB may be uninformative as patients typically have diffuse mild cortical atrophy without a clear regional pattern [34].

A meta-analysis of GM voxel-based morphometry (VBM) studies comparing clinically diagnosed PD patients with healthy controls showed greater volume loss in the medial temporal lobe and basal ganglia in PD patients. PD was associated with more severe medial temporal lobe volume loss compared with DLB. Several studies have found that patients with a clinical diagnosis of Parkinson's disease have greater atrophy than patients with Parkinson's disease without dementia [35]. Diffusion tensor imaging (DTI) often shows reduced WM integrity in PD patients [35]. DTI has shown promise as a method to differentiate AD from DLB, as clinically diagnosed DLB involves decreased fractional anisotropy (FA) in parieto-occipital WM tracts compared with AD. Several studies have found that WM in PD patients is abnormal compared with PD patients and healthy controls, as measured by FA and mean diffusivity (MD) [35].

4.3 Vascular dementia (VaD)

VaD is the third leading cause of progressive and irreversible dementia after AD (60–70%) and DLB (10–25%) [3, 4].

Due to the high variability of cerebrovascular pathological conditions and their causative factors, there are currently no universally accepted neuropathological criteria for the diagnosis of VaD. Brain pathology may show diffuse, confluent WM changes associated with age, multi-lacunar state, multiple (regional) infarcts, strategic cortical-subcortical or watershed lesions, cortical laminar necrosis (agranular cortical atrophy) delayed post-ischemic demyelination, and hippocampal sclerosis. Subcortical VaD is the most common subtype of small vessel VaD, accounting for approximately 50% of VaD cases [36]. Therefore, neuroimaging may play a key role in the diagnosis of VaD. Unlike AD, vascular diseases are classified based on morphological features rather than pathogenesis. The classification is based purely on clinical experience and does not include neuroimaging results. No criteria for establishing a causal relationship between dementia and vascular disease were mentioned [36].

The imaging manifestations of VaD can be roughly divided into (1) large vessel VaD (multi-infarct dementia, that is, multiple large complete infarcts involving cortical and subcortical areas; watershed infarcts; strategic single infarct dementia; hypoperfusion and ischemic cerebral lesions), (2) small vessel vasculopathy (subcortical vasculopathy; lacunar; perivascular spaces; silent infarcts), and (3) microbleeds and dementia (cerebral amyloid Cerebral autosomal recessive arteriopathy with subcortical infarcts and leukoencephalopathy (CADASIL); Cerebral autosomal recessive arteriopathy with subcortical infarcts and leukoencephalopathy (CARASIL); Genetic Endothelial pathology, retinopathy, nephropathy, and stroke (HERNS) [36], and the characteristics of each type are described below.

4.3.1 Large vessel VaD (LV-VaD)

Macrovascular VaD may result from multiple or single cortical or subcortical infarcts or from cerebrovascular lesions involving important areas such as the hippocampus, paramedian thalamus, and thalamocortical network. For example, vasculitis or embolism. Occlusion of the extracranial arteries, internal carotid arteries, intracranial arteries (including the middle cerebral artery), middle pial arteries, and proximal perforating arteries can lead to VaD [21, 36].

VaD depends largely on the location of the occluded vessel and the affected brain parenchyma.

Diffusion weighted imaging (DWI) and apparent diffusion coefficient (ADC) play a clear role in the diagnosis of hyperacute infarction. Infarcted areas with reduced Brownian motion appear to have restricted diffusion and have lower ADC on DWI sequences. During the subacute-chronic phase of infarction, imaging features include regional brain atrophy, gliosis, cavitation, and vacuum dilatation of the ipsilateral ventricle [36]. Encephalomalacia and gliosis are seen on T2 and fluid-attenuated inversion recovery (FLAIR) images, with loss of parenchymal tissue in the infarct area and adjacent tissues, accompanied by prominent interstitial hyperintensity in the CSF [21, 37].

Calcifications and blood product (hemosiderin) deposition may be seen on T2 and gradient echo (GRE) sequences. Corticospinal tract degeneration may also occur in hemispheric infarcts. Loss of brain tissue and its corresponding functions [36]. Left-hemisphere strokes are more frequently associated with dementia than right-hemisphere strokes. Furthermore, there was a strong association between dementia and infarctions in the left posterior cerebral artery (PCA) as well as in the anterior cerebral artery (ACA) and parietal territories. Macrophages are seen in the infarcted area with lipid-rich lamellar deposits [21]. GM is more susceptible to hypoxia than WM. On MR, laminar necrosis appears as a high-intensity signal in the cortex on T1-weighted and FLAIR images. These changes are visible within 2 weeks after infarction and are most pronounced between 1 and 3 months.

Watershed infarctions are caused by decreased blood flow or large numbers of microemboli in distal vessels. Watershed infarctions often occur at the posterior parieto-occipital junction between the cerebral arteries (PCAs) [37]. The associated hypoxia may also lead to changes in the CA-1 and CA-4 subregions of the hippocampus, the lateral halves of the caudate nucleus and putamen, and the anterior and dorsomedial nuclei of the thalamus. Generally speaking, in neuroimaging, cortical watershed infarction is manifested as a fan-shaped or wedge-shaped high signal extending from the outer edge of the lateral ventricle to the cortex, while internal watershed infarction is manifested as a high signal parallel to the lateral ventricle, but the confluence is still confluent [37]. Localized can be unilateral or bilateral.

Strategic infarct dementia is characterized by ischemic lesions in areas that control or participate in cognition and behavior or higher-order cortical functions. Thalamic stroke produces a specific form of thalamic VaD.

Aortic and cardiac disease can lead to cerebral hypoperfusion. Hypoperfusion may affect both GM and WM, with areas of hypoxia appearing at the arterial border. Hypoperfusion can also lead to hippocampal neuronal loss or severe WM changes, resulting in hippocampal sclerosis [21]. Dedicated coronal T2 and FLAIR images show a decrease in hippocampal size and an increase in signal intensity [36].

4.3.2 Small vessel VaD (SV-VaD)

MRI can more sensitively detect diffuse or localized white matter lesions (WMLs). According to the NINDS-AIREN diagnostic criteria, small vessel VaD is divided into subcortical and cortical types. Subcortical VaD (SCVD) is the most common subtype of small vessel VaD, accounting for approximately 50% of VaD cases. It is characterized by focal and diffuse ischemic WMLs, lacunar infarcts, and incomplete ischemic damage [21, 36].

Because cerebral small vessel disease (SVD) is a slowly progressive disease, prefrontal subcortical circuits are preferentially damaged. MR can reveal changes before clinical symptoms become apparent. The most common abnormality in MR is a diffuse high-intensity signal on T2-weighted imaging (T2WI), mainly occurring in the centrum semiovale, periventricular, and frontal WM [37]. On T1WI, the corresponding area may or may not show low signal. If these areas appear isointense on T1WI, they represent areas of incomplete infarction; if they appear hypointense, they are caused by complete infarction and represent tissue destruction. Vacuum dilatation of the ventricles may be seen due to periventricular leukomalacia.

The second most common imaging finding in SVD is focal WML. On T2/FLAIR images, periventricular white matter lesions (PVWMLs) can be further differentiated into smooth, well-defined hyperintensities and irregular PVWMLs. Studies have shown that dementia risk and severity of cognitive impairment are preferentially associated with PVWML, whereas mood disorders are more likely to be associated with DWML [1, 21].

Lacunar infarction refers to partial and complete infarction of a small, deep blood vessel less than 2 cm in diameter. Lacunae are most commonly found in the basal ganglia, upper two-thirds of the putamen, internal capsule, thalamus, paramedian and lateral brainstem regions, corona radiata, and centrum semiovale. MRI is more sensitive than CT for the diagnosis of acute and chronic lacunar infarction. The signal intensity of lacunar infarcts depends largely on the stage of infarction. Acute lacuna shows small areas of restricted diffusion and corresponding low ADC signal changes. In the chronic stage, these lesions appear as small round, oval, or slit-shaped cavitary infarcts ranging from a few millimeters to 1.5 cm in diameter. These lesions show high signal intensity on T2 and FLAIR images but remain low signal on T1WI [37].

The perivascular space (PVS) or Virchow–Robin space (VRS) represents the subpial interstitial space surrounding the perforating arteries and arterioles. When they are prominent in elderly patients, they indicate atrophy of the peripheral WM. Multiple enlarged VRS in the basal ganglia are called "functional subcutaneous nodules" and may clinically lead to motor impairment or cognitive decline [34]. Isointense CSF showed enhancement on all pulse sequences but not after contrast injection. They are usually bilateral and located at the level of the anterior commissure, basal ganglia, cerebral convexity, midbrain, or inferior putamen. The most common differential diagnosis is lacunar infarction, which demonstrates high signal intensity on FLAIR and proton density imaging [21, 37].

If the infarction was without stroke-like symptoms, it was defined as silent infarction. The cumulative effect of such silent infarctions may lead to cognitive deficits. Symptoms depend entirely on the damaged area and WM connections, with asymptomatic thalamic lesions having the greatest impact on memory performance. Cortical microinfarcts caused by WML and silent infarcts lead to disruption and degeneration of WM pathways connecting cortical and subcortical structures [10, 22].

4.3.3 Microbleeds and dementia (MD)

Primary massive intracerebral hemorrhage is a rare cause of dementia. Cognitive decline occurs only when the primary hemorrhage is located in critical locations such as the basal ganglia and thalamus. Microhemorrhages were defined as small, round, low-signal lesions on T2*—or susceptibility-weighted images that could not be attributed to vascular, calcified, or other pathologic causes. Microbleeds caused by sporadic

SVD are usually concentrated in the basal ganglia, and in certain locations, their distribution is mainly cortical-subcortical (lobular) [21, 36].

CAA is defined as amyloid deposition in cerebral vessels sufficient to cause vascular dysfunction. Sporadic CAA is a common cerebrovascular disease in the elderly, which is caused by the deposition of amyloid-β in the media and adventitia of the middle cerebellar artery. Vascular changes include amyloid deposition, fibrous thickening of the vessel wall, fibrinoid necrosis, and leakage of blood through the degenerated vessel wall [37].

The rapid decline in cognitive function is thought to be caused by diffuse WM changes. T2WI showed a diffuse high signal in the WM, accompanied by defects caused by ischemia. One of the main findings is the presence of multiple microhemorrhages at the epithelial-medullary junction on GRE or susceptibility-weighted imaging (SWI) images. Superficial siderosis due to cortical hemorrhage may be present. Patients may also demonstrate massive acute or subacute lobar hemorrhage on CT or MR [34].

CADASIL is a fully penetrant autosomal dominant arteriopathy. Migraines are the most common symptom. Other clinical features include transient ischemic attacks, recurrent strokes, depression, ataxia, cognitive decline, and dementia. Pathologically, the vessels showed severe arteriopathic lesions caused by deposition of granular osmophilic material in the media of small vessels, mainly involving the frontotemporal WM and lacunar infarcts, mainly in the basal ganglia.

MRI reveals two major abnormalities of CADASIL [37]: First, there are linear or punctate borders of 0.5 to 2.0 cm in the deep periventricular WM, subcortical WM, external capsule, brainstem, basal ganglia, and thalamus. Clear gaps; secondly, large areas of confluent WM changes occurred mainly in the subcortical areas of the anterior temporal and frontal lobes and involved subcortical U fibers. These changes are usually symmetrical. Band-like high signal intensity can also be seen in the external capsule, which is characteristic of CADASIL [21]. Involvement of the temporal WM, paramedian superior frontal white matter areas, and arcuate fibers is the main difference between CADASIL and Binswanger disease. MR may also demonstrate areas of low-signal intensity within dark GM nuclei on T2 and GRE images, which are thought to be caused by increased iron deposition, possibly due to disruption of axonal iron transport [36].

4.4 Frontotemporal dementia spectrum disorders (FTD)

The term FTD generally refers to three clinical syndromes, including behavioral variant frontotemporal dementia (bvFTD) and two types of Primary Progressive Aphasias (PPA), the semantic and disfluent variants of PPA. When referring to pathological entities, Frontotemporal lobar degeneration (FTLD) refers to the collection of three major pathological entities, including FTLD-tau, FTLD-TDP (TAR DNA-binding protein), and FTLD-FUS (fused in sarcomas); FTLD -Tau subtypes include corticobasal degeneration (CBD), progressive supranuclear palsy (PSP), and Pick's disease (PiD) [1, 35, 38].

4.4.1 Behavioral variant of FTD (bvFTD)

bvFTD is a neurodegenerative disorder that affects personality, behavior, and cognition. International consensus criteria for bvFTD require the presence of three of the following six symptoms in the early stages of the disease: disinhibition, apathy, loss of empathy, bulimia or change in eating habits or preferences, simple or complex repetitive movements or behaviors, and profile of poor execution in cognitive impairment.

Criteria for possible bvFTD also require frontal and/or anterior temporal lobe atrophy on MRI or CT or hypoperfusion/hypometabolism on PET or SPECT. Brain MRI can often help differentiate bvFTD from other neurodegenerative and psychiatric syndromes. Atrophy in bvFTD is common in frontotemporal structures, including the mid-insula, anterior cingulate gyrus, anterior temporal lobe, striatum, amygdala, and thalamus. However, the neuroimaging characteristics of patients with bvFTD can vary widely [35, 38].

4.4.2 Pathological basis of bvFTD and neuroimaging

The underlying pathological basis of bvFTD affects the spatial distribution of atrophy observed on brain MRI. The three common pathological substrates of bvFTD (FTLD-tau, FTLD-TDP, and FTLD-FUS) each consist of several subtypes. Tau exists in two forms resulting from alternative splicing: the three-amino acid sequence repeat form (3R) and the four-amino acid sequence repeat form (4R). The most common forms of tau associated with bvFTD are PiD (3R), CBD (4R), and PSP (4R). Each form of tau pathology is typically associated with a different pattern of atrophy. For example, PiD has asymmetric frontoinsular atrophy that extends into the anterior temporal lobes and, in severe cases, has been described as a "blade" due to severe thinning of the gyri. However, patients with bvFTD due to CBD showed relatively preserved frontoinsular regions, greater dorsal atrophy, and relative preservation of temporoparietal structures. Of note, bvFTD caused by CBD pathology is not always associated with asymmetric atrophy. Of the four subtypes of TDP-43 pathology, types A and B are most commonly associated with bvFTD syndrome. Type A is usually seen in patients with mutations in progranulin (PGRN). Type B pathology is commonly associated with FTD motor neuron disease (FTD-MND), with atrophy tending to affect the frontal lobes symmetrically with involvement of the insula and anteromedial temporal lobes. Finally, FTLD-FUS (usually sporadic) is a very rare pathological cause of bvFTD that usually presents with early onset (20 to 40 years of age) and, in addition to frontotemporal involvement, has distinct psychiatric features and severe caudate nucleus atrophy [35, 38].

4.4.3 Genetic variation and imaging

Each genetic variant of bvFTD is commonly associated with a neuroimaging phenotype. Patients with bvFTD who carry C9orf72 mutations often develop psychiatric features, including delusions. MRI in C9orf72 typically shows symmetric frontotemporal, thalamic, parietal, and cerebellar atrophy, with less medial frontal lobe atrophy compared with sporadic bvFTD. Patients with PGRN mutations exhibit a variety of clinical phenotypes, including bvFTD, nfvPPA, or CBS. In contrast to C9orf72 patients, imaging in PGRN patients often shows asymmetric frontotemporal atrophy [35, 38].

4.4.4 Corticobasal syndrome (CBS)

Consensus diagnostic criteria define CBS by early asymmetric cortical symptoms, including limb rigidity, dystonia or myoclonus, oral buccal or limb apraxia, cortical sensory deficits, and/or alien limb phenomenon. Atrophy in CBS is typically localized to the dorsal GM and WM of the posteromedial frontal and circumferential cortices as well as the basal ganglia and brainstem [38].

4.4.5 Progressive supranuclear palsies (PSPs)

The classic presentation of PSPs, often referred to as Richardson syndrome (RS), presents as atypical parkinsonism with vertical supranuclear gaze palsy or slowing of vertical saccades, as well as marked postural instability and falls. MRI in PSPs typically shows dilatation of the third ventricle, atrophy of the dorsal midbrain along the anteroposterior diameter, and atrophy of the thalamus, basal ganglia, insula, and frontal cortex [38]. Thinning of the superior cerebellar peduncles is also characteristic of this condition. Midbrain atrophy in PSPS often results in a hummingbird-like appearance of the brainstem in the sagittal plane, known as the "hummingbird" or "penguin" sign.

4.5 Prion diseases (PrD) and other rapidly progressive dementias (RPD)

RPD is defined as a condition that progresses from the first onset of symptoms to dementia in less than 2 years. Typical causes of RPD are prion diseases (PrD), including sporadic (sporadic Jacob-Creutzfeldisease, sJCD) (accounting for 85% of PrD cases), hereditary (gPrDs) (accounting for 10% of PrD cases) (10–15%) and acquired (variant). Pathological features are divided into three categories: hereditary Jacobs-Kuitzfeld disease (gJCD), Gerstmann-Straussler-Scheink (GSS), and fatal familial insomnia (FFI). It is important to note, however, that PrD does not always appear quickly. Currently, the diagnosis of PrD requires pathological examination of brain tissue. CSF testing can sometimes be helpful, but with the exception of the new reverse template earthquake-induced conversion assay (RT-QuIC), most tests are nonspecific. However, MRI is the basis for antemortem diagnosis and sometimes even helps to differentiate specific etiologies and molecular subtypes of sJCD [1, 35].

The typical neuroimaging finding associated with sJCD (and some other prion diseases) is T2/FLAIR and DWI hyperintensity in the cortex and deep GM nuclei, which can be symmetric or asymmetric, with ADC diagram. In sJCD, MRI has been shown to have higher sensitivity (91–96%) and specificity (92–94%) than almost any other diagnostic test for distinguishing JCD from other RPDs (applied to CSF and olfactory Mucosal brush test). In general, in sJCD, the GM high signal on DWI is more pronounced (brighter) than the FLAIR high signal, whereas the low signal on ADC indicates diffusion restriction [1].

DWI hyperintensity usually involves cortical and subcortical GM (68% of cases) and less commonly involves only the cortex (24%) or basal ganglia (2–5%).

Variant JCD (vJCD) often shows not only cortical involvement but also the "occipital sign," in which the occipital bone appears brighter than the anterior putamen on DWI and T2-weighted images. Sometimes, the thalamus, thalamic nuclei, and dorsomedial thalamic nuclei are all involved, resulting in the so-called hockey stick sign [1, 35]. However, these thalamic manifestations are also rare in sJCD and certain infectious and metabolic diseases such as Wernicke encephalopathy.

4.6 Idiopathic normal pressure hydrocephalus (iNPH)

iNPH is a potentially reversible cause of dementia. The clinical manifestations of this communicating hydrocephalus include the triad of cognitive impairment, gait disturbance, and urinary incontinence, as well as ventricular enlargement on neuroimaging in the presence of normal CSF pressure [1].

The diagnosis of iNPH is important because it is one of the few forms of dementia that can be treated, if not reversed, if caught early.

Two imaging diagnostic indicators, Evans index (EI) and callosal angle (CA), are often used as first-line quantitative indicators of ventricular enlargement in iNPH on cross-sectional imaging. EI (defined as the ratio between the widest diameter of the frontal horn and the maximum internal diameter of the skull measured in the same axial plane) is a commonly used parameter to quantify ventriculomegaly, although this ratio varies depending on the position and angle of the frontal horn. International guidelines recommend a threshold of 0.3, while some authors recommend a more stringent threshold of 0.33. EI is not specific to iNPH and is increased in patients with atrophy. CA helps differentiate iNPH from vacuum hydrocephalus. It is measured in the coronal plane at the posterior commissure perpendicular to the anterior/posterior commissure (AC-PC) plane. Patients with iNPH generally have a smaller angle of 50–80° compared to patients with hydrocephalus (100–120°) [38].

4.7 Cerebellar diseases

Multiple System Atrophy (MSA) is a progressive neurodegenerative disease characterized pathologically by widespread α-synuclein-positive glial cytoplasmic inclusions in the striatonigral and/or olivopontocerebellar regions. Clinically, MSA presents with a combination of progressive autonomic failure and motor symptoms. When motor symptoms include Parkinson's syndrome that does not respond well to levodopa, it is called MSA-Parkinson syndrome or (MSA-P). When the prominent motor feature is cerebellar, the syndrome is called MSA-cerebellar (MSA-C).

MSA-C usually displays the classic "hot cross bun" (HCB) or "cruciform T2" sign, which is characterized by pontine hyperintensity on axial T2/FLAIR and/or proton density-weighted MRI. This sign helps differentiate MSA from other Parkinsonian syndromes. Several studies have demonstrated significantly greater striatal, brainstem, and cerebellar atrophy in MSA compared with PD and PSP [35, 38].

4.8 Inherited neurological diseases

Inherited neurological disorders are generally relatively uncommon. Inheritance follows the basic Mendelian laws of somatic dominant, somatic recessive, and X-linked recessive inheritance.

4.8.1 Neurofibromatosis type 1 (NFT1)

Neurofibromatosis type 1 is an autosomal dominant disorder with age-dependent penetrance caused by defects in the NF1 gene (neurofibromin) on chromosome 17q, with a frequency of approximately 1 in 4–5000. Clinically, it is characterized by neurofibromas on peripheral nerves, multiple dermatofibromas, and more than five pigmented or café-au-lait spots (CAL) on the trunk. Clinical manifestations can range from few to numerous and distinctive skin lesions. Other clinical findings include axillary, neck, and groin freckles, Lisch nodules on the iris, and sometimes scoliosis. Patients with type 1 may develop paraplegia secondary to enlarging intraaxial neurofibromas due to nerve root compression of the spinal cord [35].

4.8.2 Neurofibromatosis type 2 (NFT2)

Neurofibromatosis type 2 is a very rare somatically dominant genetic disorder that affects approximately 1 in 50,000 people due to a defect in the NF2 gene (Merlin) on chromosome 22. They are intracranial tumors, acoustic neuromas (vestibular schwannoma), and meningiomas. The main clinical manifestation of type 2 is deafness caused by an acoustic neuroma involving the eighth cranial nerve. Although acoustic neuromas are usually bilateral on neuroimaging, clinical features at presentation are often unilateral. The diagnosis is usually confirmed by MRI [35].

4.8.3 Tuberous sclerosis

It is an autosomal dominant disorder caused by mutations in TSC1 (hammerin) on chromosome 9q or TSC2 (potatocin) on chromosome 16p, with a prevalence of 1/15,000. The main clinical features are characteristic facial angiofibromatous or adenomatous sebaceous lesions on the cheeks and nose, together with a history of epilepsy. There may be associated cognitive impairment. Other cutaneous manifestations include ash hypopigmented macular plaques and sharkskin plaques, which are 1–10 cm orange peel-like subepidermal fibrotic plaques that most commonly occur in the lumbosacral region and subungual fibromas. CT shows a characteristic pattern of paraventricular subependymal calcified nodules or nodules [35].

4.8.4 Spinocerebellar disorders (SCA)

SCA is an autosomal dominant, clinically diverse neurodegenerative disorder characterized by progressive cerebellar ataxia, sometimes with other concomitant signs and/or symptoms. Although all SCAs may present with a cerebellar phenotype accompanied by cerebellar atrophy, a few have additional clinical and neuroimaging findings. Classic CT or MRI in SCA patients shows only cerebellar atrophy [35].

4.8.5 Hereditary neuropathy

These are also called hereditary motor sensory neuropathies (HMSN). Peroneal muscular atrophy (CMT1 = HMSN1) or peroneal muscular atrophy is the most common clinical example. It is an autosomal dominant disorder primarily due to a 1, 5 Mb duplication involving the PMP22 gene on chromosome 17p. It affects about 1/3000 people, with marked muscle atrophy of the lower legs and distal thighs, accompanied by bilateral pes cavus (high cavus, claw-like toes) and loss of reflexes [1, 34, 35].

4.8.6 Huntington's disease (HD)

HD is an autosomal dominant neurodegenerative disorder that presents with choreiform movements, progressive dementia, and psychiatric symptoms in midlife. Caused by a trinucleotide repeat expansion of the CAG in the huntingtin gene on chromosome 4, it results in progressive motor, cognitive, and behavioral dysfunction. The most consistently reported structural neuroimaging finding in HD is striatal atrophy [1, 34, 35]. In the overt (motor) phase of HD, structural MRI typically shows global volume loss throughout the brain, basal ganglia, brainstem, and cerebellum, although the caudate, putamen, nucleus accumbens, and amygdala remain the most atrophied [1, 34, 35, 38].

4.8.7 Muscle diseases

The main genetic myopathies are dystrophies, Duchenne muscular dystrophy (DMD), Becker muscular dystrophy (BMD), limb-girdle muscular dystrophy (LGMD), facioscapulohumeral muscular dystrophy (FSHD), and myotonic dystrophy bad [34].

4.8.8 Hereditary spastic paraplegia (HSP)

This is a rare hereditary form of spastic paraplegia that usually follows an autosomal dominant inheritance pattern and less commonly recessive and X-linked inheritance. Multiple genetic mutations involve more than 20 different sites on different chromosomes, with spasticity gene mutations on chromosome 2p22 accounting for 40–50% of cases. The most common clinical phenotype is usually slowly progressive spastic paraplegia starting in childhood or adolescence, characterized by hyperreflexia and toe-up, with progressively increasing difficulty walking [34].

4.8.9 Wilson's disease (WD)

Wilson's disease is an autosomal recessive disorder of copper metabolism with neurological and hepatic symptoms. Chelation therapy is used in "decoppered" patients, but the neurological outcome remains unpredictable. A range of neuroimaging abnormalities have been described that may provide insights into disease mechanisms in addition to prognostic and monitoring biomarkers. Previous quantitative MRI analyzes have focused on specific sequences or regions of interest, often stratifying chronically treated patients based on ongoing symptoms rather than initial presentation. When comparing patients with neurological and hepatic manifestations, GM volumes are lower in the basal ganglia, thalamus, brainstem, cerebellum, anterior insula, and orbitofrontal cortex [1, 34, 39, 40]. In stable patients under long-term

Disease	Cause	Symptoms	neuroimaging features/Damage area	Corresponding neuroimaging
AD	Abnormal aggregation of beta-amyloid and tau proteins.	Cognitive impairment	Early atrophy of the hippocampus and precuneus. SPECT images show reduced regional cerebral blood flow.	**Figure 16**
DLB & PD	Neurodegeneration	Decreased visual function and amnesia	Diffuse mild cortical atrophy, medial temporal lobe and basal ganglia volume loss, and reduced white matter integrity.	**Figure 17**
LV-VaD	Cortical or subcortical infarction, cerebrovascular disease, vasculitis, or embolism.	Stroke, dementia	Local brain atrophy, gliosis, and ventricular vacuum dilatation. Marked cerebrospinal fluid (CSF) spaces. Sclerosis and reduction in size of the hippocampus.	**Figure 18**

Disease	Cause	Symptoms	neuroimaging features/Damage area	Corresponding neuroimaging
SV-VaD	Focal and diffuse ischemic WML, lacunar infarction, and incomplete ischemic injury.	Stroke, dementia, mood disorders, cognitive impairment.	Periventricular leukomalacia and ventricular vacuum dilatation. Lacunar infarction. Multiple punctate or confluent lesions in the white matter. Microbleeds.	**Figure 19**
MD	Beta-amyloid deposition in the media and adventitia of the middle cerebellar artery.	Rapid decline in cognitive function, migraine, cerebral ischemia, recurrent stroke, depression, ataxia, dementia.	Diffuse white matter hyperintensities, confluent white matter changes occur primarily in subcortical regions of the anterior temporal and frontal lobes and involve subcortical U fibers.	**Figure 20**
bvFTD	Frontal island & caudate nucleus atrophy.	Bulimia, repetitive movements, cognitive impairment.	Frontal insula and caudate nucleus atrophy.	**Figure 21**
CBS	Cortical atrophy	Dystonia, cortical sensory deficits, alien limb phenomenon.	Left frontal lobe atrophy, temporoparietal atrophy.	**Figure 22**
PSPs	The dorsal midbrain atrophies along the anterior–posterior diameter, and the thalamus, basal ganglia, insula, and frontal cortex atrophy.	Vertical supranuclear gaze palsy falls.	Midbrain area is reduced. Thinning of superior cerebellar peduncle. Hummingbird-like appearance of the brainstem in the sagittal plane.	**Figure 23**
PPA	Atrophy occurs in discrete locations in the brain.	svPPA、nfvPPA、lvPPA	Brain atrophy, GM loss, volume loss in the middle temporal gyrus, and angular gyrus.	**Figure 24**
RPD	Prion disease	Dementia	The occiput appears brighter than the anterior putamen. Hockey stick logo. Cerebellar atrophy.	**Figure 25**
iNPH	Ventricular enlargement	Cognitive impairment, gait impairment, and urinary incontinence.	Ventricular enlargement.	**Figure 26**
MSA	Neurodegeneration. Misfolded alpha-synuclein.	Progressive autonomic failure.	Pontine hyperintensity. Extensive alpha-synuclein-positive glial cytoplasmic inclusions.	**Figure 27**
SCA	Somatic chromosomal dominant inheritance, neurodegeneration.	progressive cerebellar ataxia	Chronic cerebellar degeneration.	**Figure 28**

Disease	Cause	Symptoms	neuroimaging features/Damage area	Corresponding neuroimaging
HD	Trinucleotide repeat expansion of CAG in the huntingtin gene on chromosome 4.	Progressive motor, cognitive, and behavioral dysfunction.	Striatum atrophy. Whole brain volume loss.	**Figure 29**
NFT 1	NF1 gene defect on chromosome 17q.	Paraplegia.	Neurofibromas on peripheral nerves, multiple dermatofibromas, and more than five pigmented macules on the trunk.	**Figure 30**
NFT2	Defects in the NF2 gene (Merlin) on chromosome 22.	Deaf.	Acoustic neuroma. Schwannomas are heterogeneous in intensity on T2-weighted sequences. Post-gadolinium T1-weighted sequences were significantly enhanced.	**Figure 31**
Tuberous sclerosis	TSC1 on chromosome 9q or TSC2 mutation on chromosome 16p.	Angiofibroma, cognitive impairment, macular hypopigmentation spots, and shark skin spots.	Paraventricular subependymal calcified nodules. Cortical or subependymal nodules and white matter abnormalities. Renal angiomyolipoma. Cardiac rhabdomyomas.	**Figure 32**
HMSN	Due to 1, 5 Mb duplication involving the PMP22 gene on chromosome 17p.	The distal calf and thigh muscles were significantly atrophied.	Optic atrophy.	**Figure 33**
muscle disease	Malnutrition	DMD, BMD, LGMD, FSHD, and myotonic muscular dystrophy.	The calf muscles showed symmetrical atrophy and fatty infiltration.	**Figure 34**
HSP	Multiple genetic mutations involved.	Slowly progressive spastic paraplegia.	Cerebellar, optic atrophy, peripheral neuropathy, eye palsy, macular degeneration. The corpus callosum is thin. Shows the typical "lynx ears" sign on FLAIR sequences.	**Figure 35**
WD	A deficiency of ceruloplasmin in the blood.	Cirrhosis of the liver, copper deposits on the cornea.	Basal ganglia lesions. Showing "bright claustrum." Signal intensity increased bilaterally in the globus pallidus and midbrain.	**Figure 36**

Table 7.
Neuroimaging characteristics of specific neurological diseases.

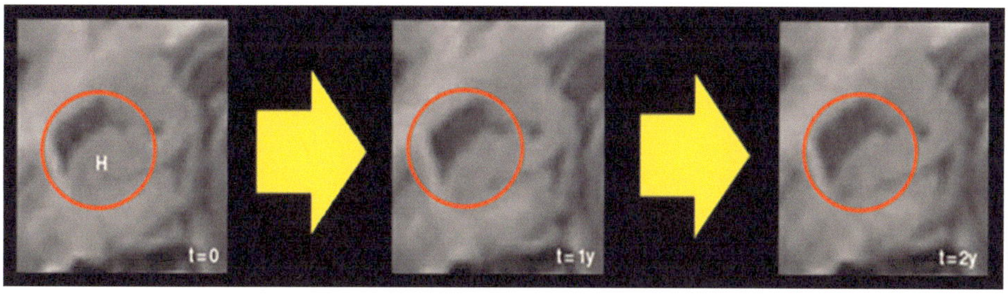

Figure 16.
Annual T1-weighted studies of AD patients show progressive hippocampal shrinkage.

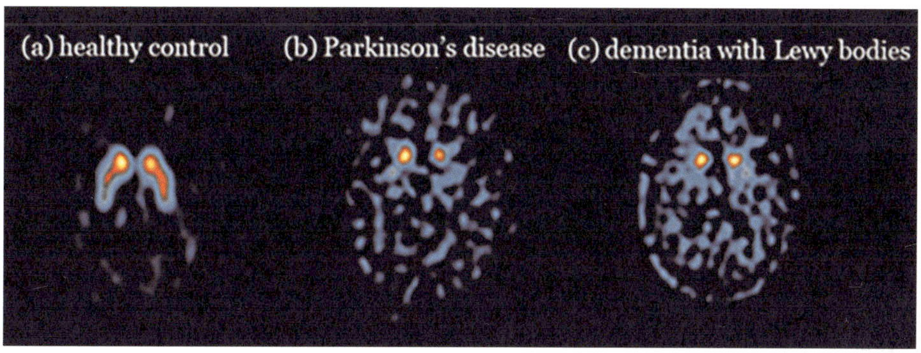

Figure 17.
Application of DaTSCAN (FP-CIT) in patients with Parkinson's disease and Lewy body dementia.

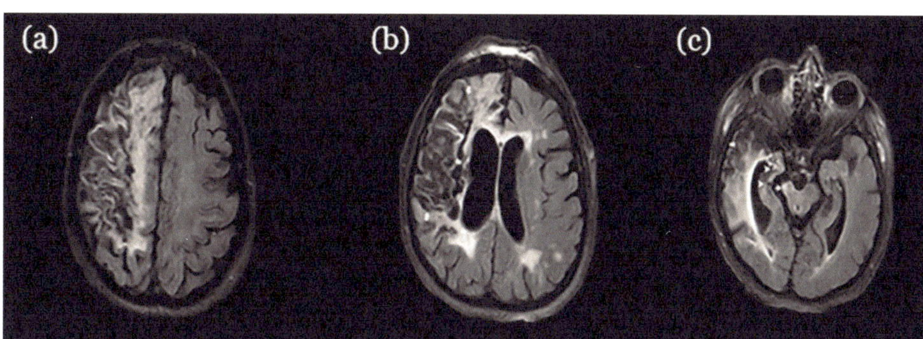

Figure 18.
Axial FLAIR MR image showed a large chronic infarct in the right MCA with peripheral hyperintensity due to cerebral softening and gliosis.

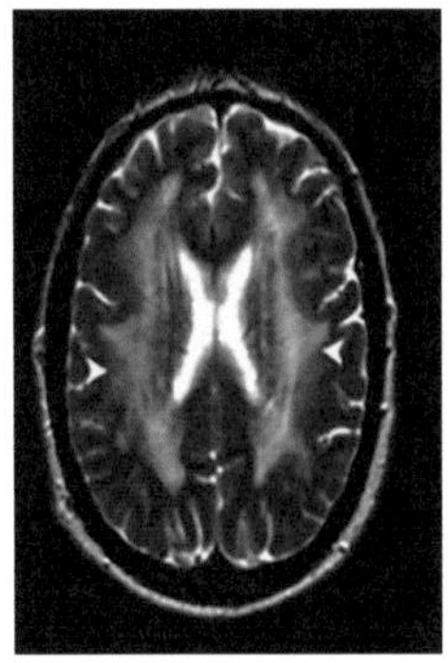

Figure 19.
Diffuse SVD accompanies subcortical dementia.

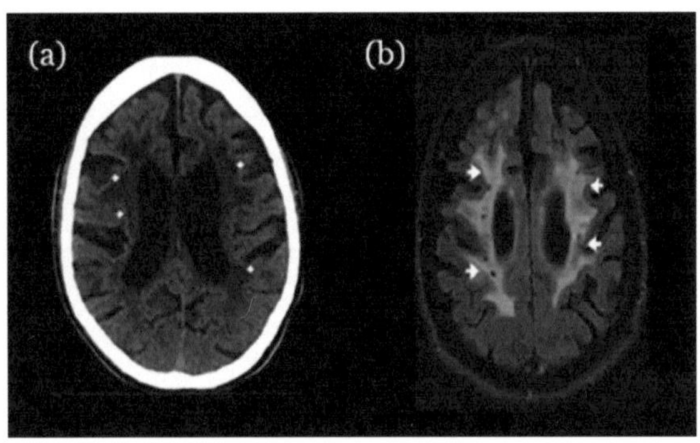

Figure 20.
Cerebral amyloid angiopathy.

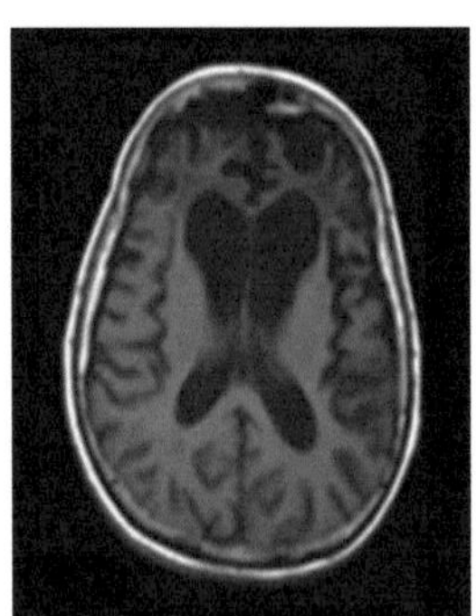

Figure 21.
Frontal cortical and white matter atrophy in patients with frontotemporal dementia.

DOI: http://dx.doi.org/10.5772/intechopen.1009347

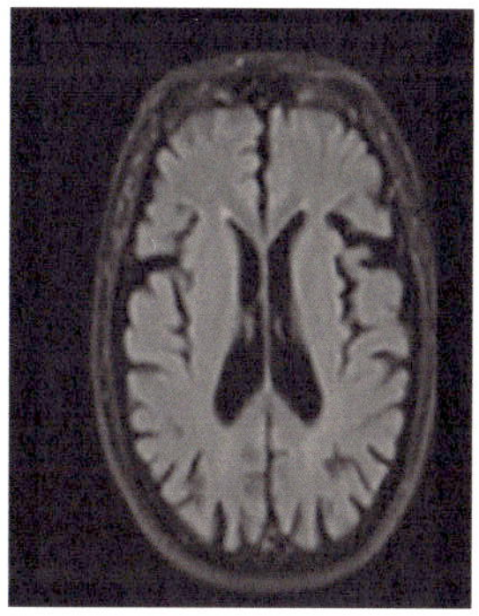

Figure 22.
A patient with CBS had bilateral frontotemporal and parietal cortical atrophy.

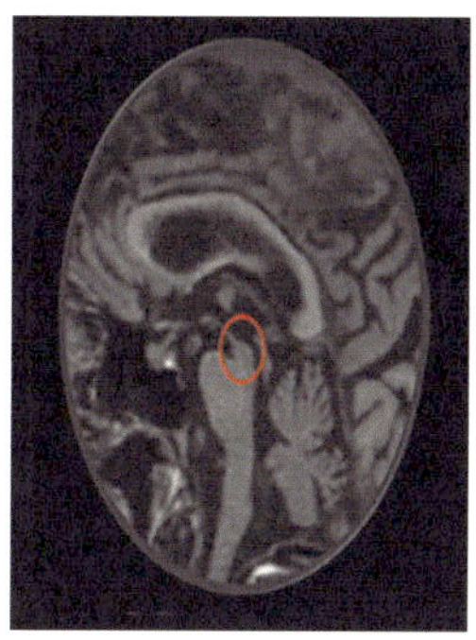

Figure 23.
A patient with FTLD-PSP had a significantly smaller area of the brain.

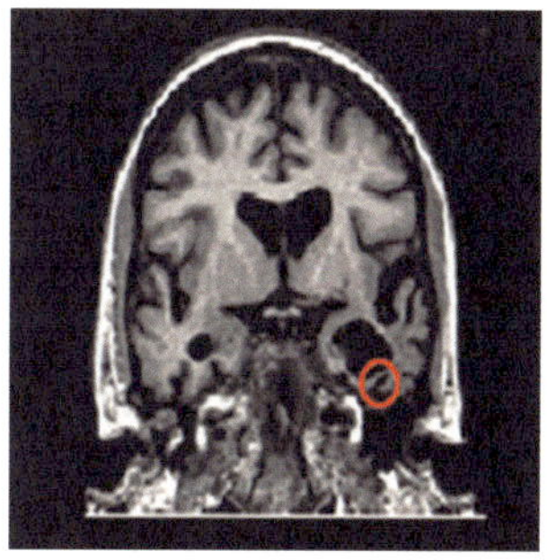

Figure 24.
A patient with svPPA had the most pronounced atrophy in the left cleft.

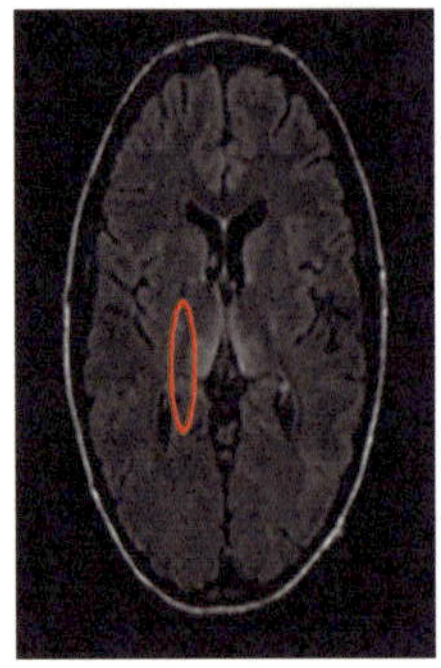

Figure 25.
A patient with a JCD variant had a pincushion sign.

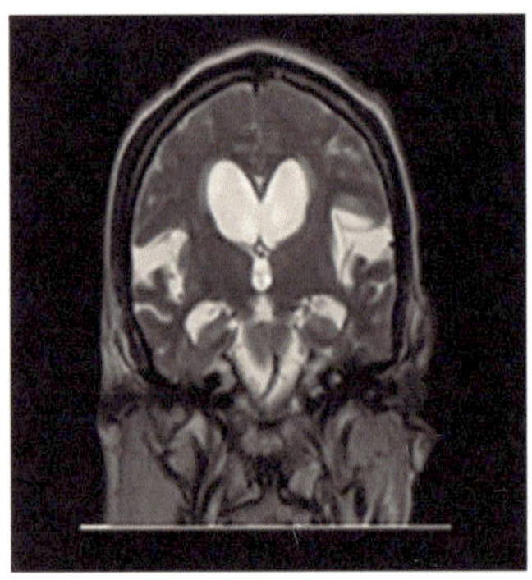

Figure 26.
A patient with iNPH have significantly enlarged ventricles.

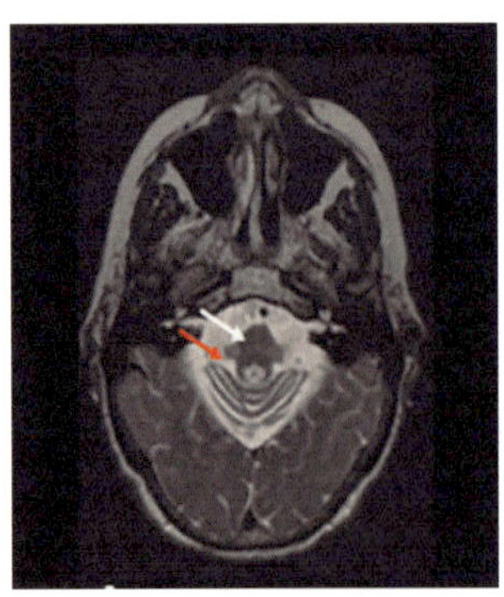

Figure 27.
High signal at MCP junction in patients with MSA-C.

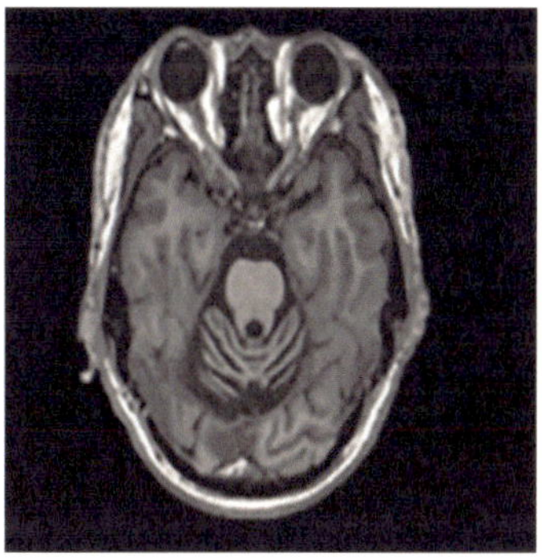

Figure 28.
Characteristics of chronic cerebellar degeneration in a SCAR16 patient.

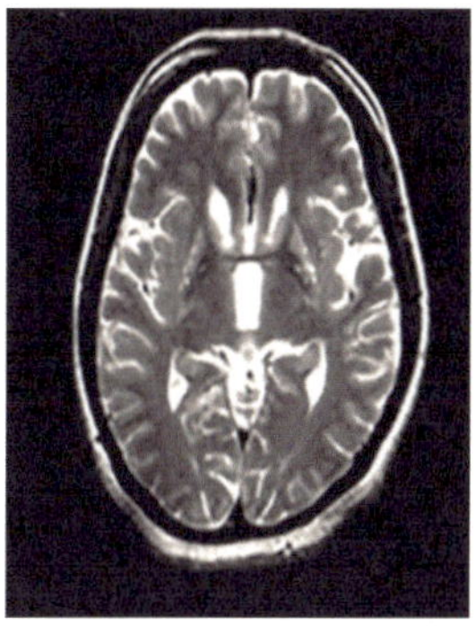

Figure 29.
Bilateral striatum atrophy and degeneration in a patient with HD.

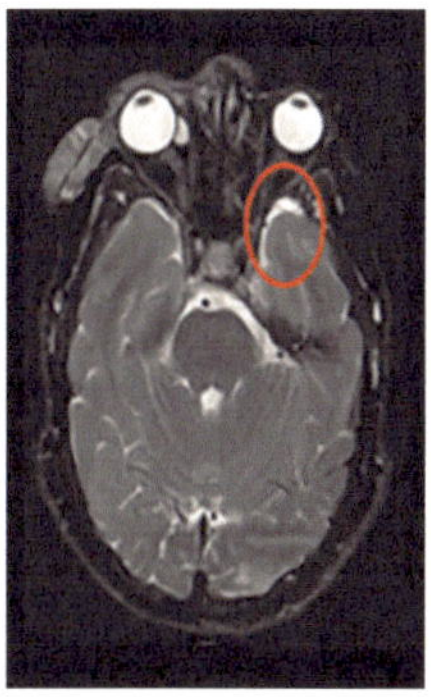

Figure 30.
Left optic nerve glioma.

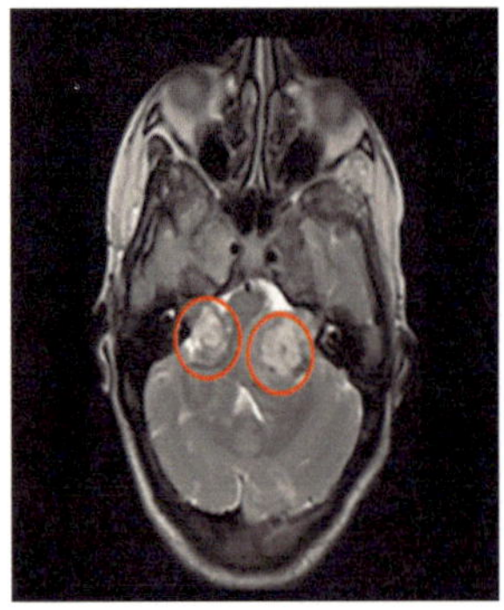

Figure 31.
Schwannomas have heterogeneous intensity.

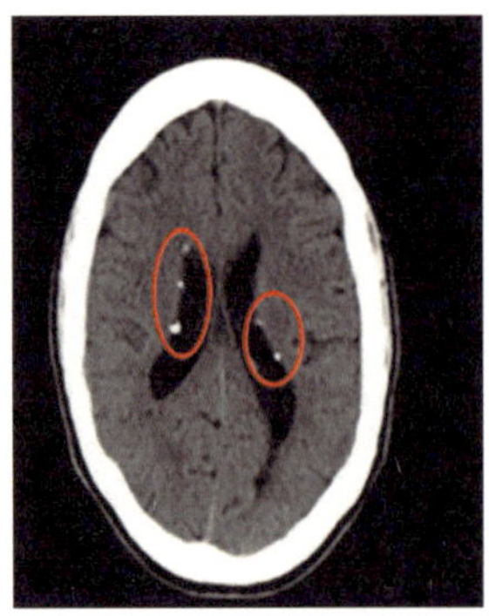

Figure 32.
Subependymal nodule in a patient with tuberous sclerosis.

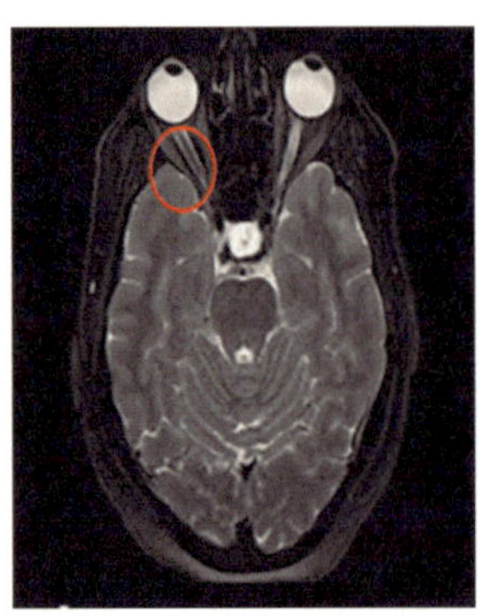

Figure 33.
A patient with HMSN have an abnormally thin and reduced size of the left optic nerve.

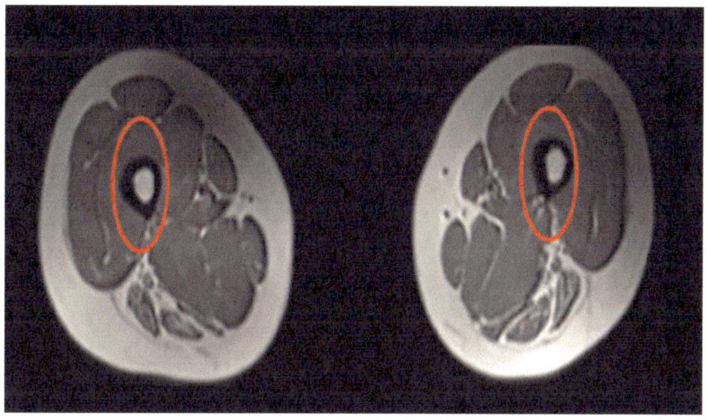

Figure 34.
Symmetric atrophy and fatty infiltration of the hamstrings inpatients with muscle disease.

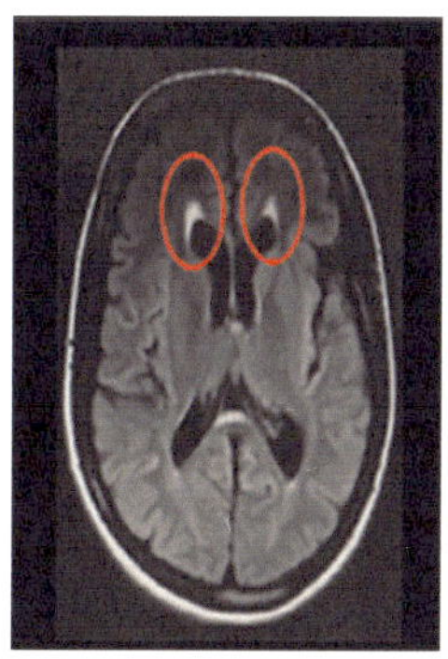

Figure 35.
Typical "lynx ears" sign on FLAIR sequence of HSP patients.

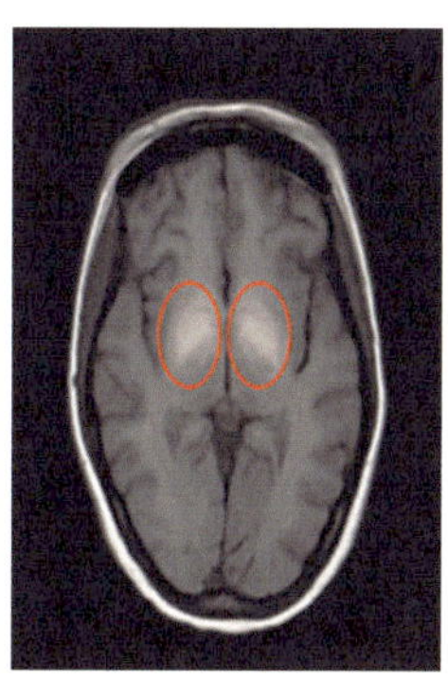

Figure 36.
T1-weighted axial MR image shows increased signal intensity in the globus pallidus.

treatment, the severity of neurological deficits is associated with similar, predominantly subcortical, GM volumes [39, 40].

Regarding the content mentioned in this section, the characteristics of neuroimaging corresponding to special neurological diseases are compiled as shown in **Table** 7 and **Figures 16–36**.

5. Conclusions and suggestions

Currently, there are still few studies that summarize the neuroimaging features corresponding to neurological diseases. Sobański et al. [41] proposed MRI image features for identifying diseases including PSP, MSA, CBD, Creutzfeldt-Jakob disease (CJD), WD, and CADASIL (**Figure 37**), which can be used to visually distinguish the typical features of these diseases, thereby assisting neurologists and neuroradiologists make the decisions. Chang et al. [42] have also summarized the clinical data on stroke, dural vein thrombosis, arterial dissection, vasculitis, and intraparenchymal.

Neurological imaging characteristics and diseases affected by neurological diseases such as hemorrhage, PRES, leukoencephalopathy, and cranial neuropathy.

This chapter collects neuroimaging features in order to obtain conclusions that can help doctors improve the level, convenience, and accuracy of clinical diagnosis. Sections 3 and 4 summarize the neuroimaging features of somatic neurological injuries and selected chronic/genetic neurological disorders. According to **Tables 6** and 7, physical nerve damage can be found. The location of nerve damage can be easily

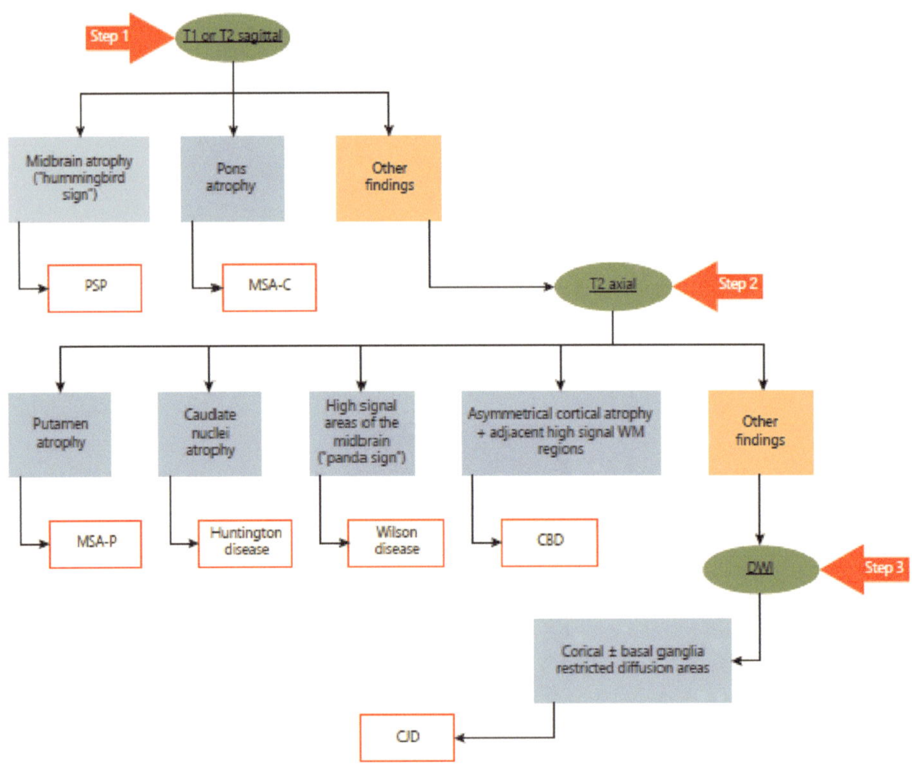

Figure 37.
A practical approach to imaging findings on conventional MRI in suspected neurodegenerative disease [42].

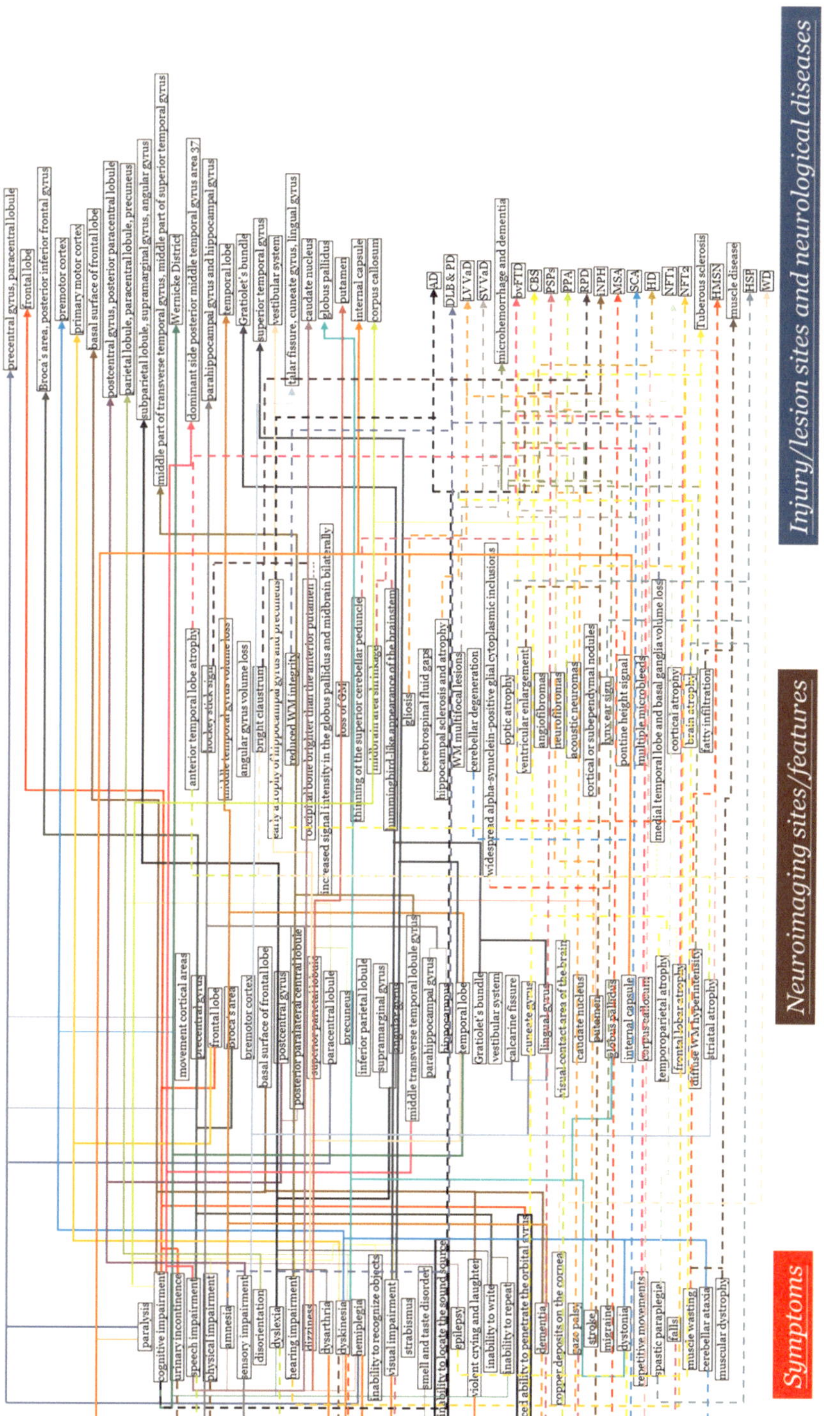

Figure 38.
Nervous system diseases and neuroimaging feature retrieval map.

determined by the symptoms of language disorders, visual disorders, and movement disorders. However, chronic neurological diseases must be assisted by neuroimaging. In order to diagnose the disease more accurately, since most chronic neurological diseases have symptoms of dementia, the importance of neuroimaging-assisted diagnosis is highlighted. At the end of this chapter, the symptoms and neuroimaging features of common neurological diseases are summarized and made into a search map (**Figure 38**). When using it, we must first determine the possible site of nerve damage based on the patient's symptoms and medical history, then use the most accurate neuroimaging technology to detect the disease and confirm the disease based on the results.

The final suggestion of this chapter is that if reconfirmation can be performed through two or more neuroimaging techniques, the accuracy of physicians' clinical diagnosis can be greatly improved. In the future, clinicians will be able to quickly and accurately diagnose the disease based on the symptoms and neuroimaging shown in **Figure 38**.

Author details

Tse Jung Liu
Graduate Institute of Environmental Engineering, National Taiwan University, Taipei, Taiwan

*Address all correspondence to: argus0327@gmail.com

References

[1] Kato JK. Advancements in neuroimaging for early detection of neurological disorders. EEJPH. 2024; **5**(2):2992-4081

[2] Vemuri P, Jack Jr CR. Role of structural MRI in Alzheimer's disease. Vemuri and Jack Jr Alzheimer's Research & Therapy. 2010;**2**:23

[3] Jack CR, Barnesb J, Bernstein MA, et al. Magnetic resonance imaging in Alzheimer's disease neuroimaging initiative 2. Alzheimer's & Dementia. 2015;**11**:740-756

[4] Park M, Moon W-J. Structural MR imaging in the diagnosis of Alzheimer's disease and other neurodegenerative dementia: Current imaging approach and future perspectives. Korean Journal of Radiology. 2016;**17**(6):827-845

[5] Symms M, Jager HR, Schmierer K, Yousry TA. A review of structural magnetic resonance neuroimaging. Journal of Neurology, Neurosurgery, and Psychiatry. 2004;**75**:1235-1244

[6] Noh J-H, Kim J-H, Yang H-D. Classification of Alzheimer's progression using fMRI data. Sensors. 2023;**23**:6330

[7] Torres AL. Neuroimaging biomarkers for early diagnosis of Alzheimer's disease. An approach from neural networks. Revista chilena de radiologica. 2020;**26**(3):105-112

[8] Warren SL, Moustafa AA. Functionalmagnetic resonance imaging, deep learning, and Alzheimer's disease: A systematic review. Journal of Neuroimaging. 2023;**33**:5-18

[9] Kim JH, Jeong M, Stiles WR, Choi HS. Neuroimaging modalities in Alzheimer's disease: Diagnosis and clinical features. International Journal of Molecular Sciences. 2022;**23**:6079

[10] Masdeu JC, Gadhia R, Faridar A. Brain CT and MRI: Differential diagnosis of imaging findings. In: Handbook of Clinical Neurology. Vol. 136. Cambridge, MA: Elsevier; 2016. pp. 1037-1054

[11] Perillo T, Capasso R, Pinto A. Neuroimaging of the most common meningitis and encephalitis of adults: A narrative review. Diagnostics. 2024;**14**: 1064

[12] Raji CA, Tarzwell R, Pavel D, Schneider H, Uszler M, Thornton J, et al. Clinical utility of SPECT neuroimaging in the diagnosis and treatment of traumatic brain injury: A systematic review. PLoS One. 2014;**9**(3):1-10

[13] Arbizua J, García-Ribasb G, Carrióc I, et al. Recommendations for the use of PET imaging biomarkers in the diagnosis of neurodegenerative conditions associated with dementia: Consensus proposal from the SEMNIM and SEN. Revista Espanola De Medicina Nuclear E Imagen Molecular. 2015;**34**(5): 303-313

[14] Ozsahin I, Sekeroglu B, Mok GSP. The use of back propagation neural networks and 18F-Florbetapir PET for early detection of Alzheimer's disease using Alzheimer's disease neuroimaging initiative database. PLoS One. 2019;**14**(12):e0226577

[15] Ricci M, Cimini A, Chiaravalloti A, Filippi L, Schillaci O. Positron emission tomography (PET) and neuroimaging in the personalized approach to neurodegenerative causes of dementia. International Journal of Molecular Sciences. 2020;**21**:7481

[16] Bazira PJ. An overview of the nervous system. Surgery (Oxford). 2021; **39**(8):451-462

[17] Knight J, Bayram-Weston Z, Andrade-Sienz M. Nervous system 1: Introduction to the nervous system. In: Systems of Life. London: Nursing Times; 2022

[18] Michel LC, McCormick EM, Kievit RA. Gray and white matter metrics demonstrate distinct and complementary prediction of differences in cognitive performance in children: Findings from ABCD (N = 11,876). The Journal of Neuroscience. 2024;**44**(12): e0465232023

[19] Giovannoni F, Quintana FJ. The role of astrocytes in CNS inflammation. Trends in Immunology. 2020;**41**:805-819

[20] Wang R, Ren H, Gao Y, Wang G. Editorial: Role of glial cells of the central and peripheral nervous system in the pathogenesis of neurodegenerative disorders. Frontiers in Aging Neuroscience. 2022;**14**:920861

[21] Kiefer J, Mazzeffi M. Complications of vascular disease. Anesthesiology Clinics. 2022;**40**:587-604

[22] Friedman MJ, Resick PA, Bryant RA, et al. Classification of trauma and stressor-related disorders in DSM-5. Depression and Anxiety. 2011;**28**: 737-749

[23] Savoiardo M, Grisoli M. Degenerative diseases. In: Demaerel P, editor. Recent Advances in Diagnostic Neuroradiology. Medical Radiology. Berlin, Heidelberg: Springer; 2001

[24] Patel A. Benign vs malignant tumors. JAMA Oncology. 2020;**6**(9):1488

[25] Heinasmaki T, Fawcett-Henesy A. Infections and Infectious Diseases. Geneve Switzerland: WHO; 2001

[26] Koppala SN, Guruprasad V. Overview of autoimmunity: Classification, disease mechanisms, and etiolog. Turkish Journal of Immunology. 2023;**11**(3):93-105

[27] Kimberley TJ, Lewis SM. Understanding Neuroimaging. Physical Therapy. 2007;**87**(6):670-683

[28] Aiken AH. Central nervous system infection. Neuroimaging Clinics of North America. 2010;**20**:557-580

[29] John DM, Danielle SB. Network Analyses and Nervous System Disorders. arXiv:1701.01101v1 [q-bio.NC] 4; 2017. Hall Ithaca, NY: arXiv, Engineering Library Carpenter;

[30] Chételat G, Arbizu J, Barthel H, et al. Amyloid-PET and ^{18}F-FDG-PET in the diagnostic investigation of Alzheimer's disease and other dementias. Lancet Neurology. 2020;**19**:951-962

[31] Bao W, Xie F, Zuo C. Guan Y and Huang YH PET neuroimaging of Alzheimer's disease: Radiotracers and their utility in clinical research. Frontiers in Aging Neuroscience. 2021;**13**: 624330

[32] Khalafi M, Rashnoudi AR, et al. Amyloid PET scan diagnosis of Alzheimer's disease in patients with multiple sclerosis: A scoping review study. Egyptian Journal of Radiology and Nuclear Medicine. 2023;**54**:12

[33] Chang-Hsien O, Liu T-J, Cheng C-S, Lin P-L, Lee C-L. Neuroimaging for early diagnosis of Alzheimer's disease: A review. Clinical Laboratory. 2024;**70**: 1055-1068

[34] Roelofs JJ, Teodoro T, Edwards MJ. Neuroimaging in functional movement disorders. Current Neurology and Neuroscience Reports. 2019;**19**:12

[35] Staffaroni AM, Elahi FM, McDermott D, Marton K, Karageorgiou E, Sacco S, et al. Neuroimaging in dementia. Seminars in Neurology. 2017;**37**:510-537

[36] Kanekar S, Poot JD. Neuroimaging of vascular dementia. Radiologic Clinics of North America. 2014;**52**:383-401

[37] Heiss W-D. Neuroimaging in cerebral small vessel disease. Journal of Neurology and Neuromedicine. 2018; **3**(2):1-7

[38] Howlett WP. Inherited Neurological Disorders. Oslo, Norway: BRIC; 2012

[39] Ma X-f, Fan L-y, Jin P, Lin K, Tong G-a, Wang G-q. Clinical and neuroimaging features in neurological Wilson's disease with claustrum lesions. Scientific Reports. 2024;**14**:22266

[40] Patel K, Bhayana A, Bagri N, Malik A. Case series on neuroimaging spectrum of Wilson's disease: Knowing the known and the uncommonly known. Egyptian Journal of Radiology and Nuclear Medicine. 2024;**55**:157

[41] Sobański M, Zacharzewska-Gondek A, Waliszewska-Prosół M, et al. A review of neuroimaging in rare neurodegenerative diseases. Dementia and Geriatric Cognitive Disorders. 2020; **49**:544-556

[42] Chang S, Schecht M, Jain R, Belani P. Acute neurological complications of coronavirus disease. Neuroimaging Clinics of North America. 2023;**33**:57-68

Chapter 3

Functional Neuroimaging in Nuclear Medicine

Nur Aydinbelge Dizdar and Derya Cayir

Abstract

Nuclear medicine imaging modalities are frequently used as highly sensitive disease markers and clinical application tools in the evaluation and diagnosis of dementia and movement disorders that develop due to neurodegenerative pathological processes in the brain. In epilepsy, nuclear medicine imaging modalities are used in ictal and/or interictal periods to determine the epileptic focus before surgical intervention in drug-resistant epilepsy. Brain death scan with parenchymal radiopharmaceuticals plays an important role in patient management as it provides the opportunity to evaluate both the brain and the brainstem. Currently, PET imaging modalities are employed to differentiate between primary central nervous system tumors and metastatic lesions, to assess treatment response and to guide biopsy.

Keywords: nuclear medicine, SPECT, PET, radiopharmaceuticals, dementia, movement disorders, epilepsy, brain death scan, brain tumors

1. Introduction

This chapter initiates with an overview of the major neuroimaging modalities and their importance in the diagnosis of brain disorders. It then explores the specific applications of MRI, CT, and US in neuroimaging, highlighting their advantages and limitations. The discussion then moves on to molecular imaging techniques such as PET/CT and SPECT/CT, emphasizing their role in the assessment of neurodegenerative diseases, epilepsy, and another neuropsychiatric conditions. The chapter concludes by examining the integration of neuroimaging in the diagnosis and management of brain tumors, as well as the potential impact of future innovations in imaging technologies and radiopharmaceuticals.

Neuroimaging modalities have an important role in the management of brain disorders, providing a precise diagnosis or clinically relevant differential diagnoses because there are many etiologies leading to neuropathology, including vascular, infectious-inflammatory, degenerative, and neoplastic entities whose clinical signs and symptoms are often non-specific. The anatomical imaging modalities such as cranial ultrasonography (US), computed tomography (CT), and magnetic resonance (MRI) and the hybrid imaging modalities such as single-photon emission computed tomography (SPECT) combined with computed tomography (SPECT/CT) and positron emission tomography (PET) combined with computed tomography (PET/CT) are currently available neuroimaging modalities, each with its own strengths and limitations.

 IntechOpen

Generally, MRI is the most useful technique for examining the brain due to its higher soft tissue contrast, but CT still has an essential role in emergency imaging and is also the best technique for examining associated bony structures. Furthermore, functional MRI (fMRI) is a type of MRI scan that can demonstrate time-varying changes in brain metabolism by detecting changes associated with regional blood flow. Cranial US has a vital role in fetal and neonatal imaging due to its ease and the presence of the skull foramina, which is a good acoustic window in this population.

The molecular imaging modalities PET/CT and SPECT/CT are widely used in daily routine to obtain functional and anatomical information. Particularly, PET imaging with ^{18}F-fluoro-2-deoxy-d-glucose (FDG PET) has become a cornerstone in the evaluation of neurodegenerative diseases such as Alzheimer's disease (AD), frontotemporal dementia (FTD), and dementia with Lewy body (DLB), assisting diagnosis, staging, and management. Brain SPECT and planar imaging have been applied in the evaluation of various neurological and psychiatric disorders, including dementia, epilepsy, movement disorders, cerebrovascular disease, and psychiatric conditions. It provides the visualization and quantification of regional cerebral blood flow (rCBF) and density studies.

Neuroimaging methods have a crucial role in diagnosis and post-treatment evaluation of brain tumors, contributing to treatment optimization, prognosis, and patient management. Hybrid molecular imaging modalities with various radiopharmaceuticals provide important information about brain tumors and other areas of the body, including the metabolism, physiology, and functionality of the tumor. Nuclear medicine imaging modalities will become even more important in clinical use if further innovations in imaging techniques and radiopharmaceuticals help to diagnose neurological disorders at an early stage.

2. SPECT and SPECT/CT imaging

SPECT is an imaging method in which three-dimensional functional images of brain regions are obtained after administered of a gamma photon emitting radiopharmaceutical has properties such as distribution according to cerebral perfusion, neurotransmitter or cell density by crossing the blood–brain barrier (**Table 1**). Brain perfusion imaging with HMPAO and ECD and the cerebral receptor binding agents ^{123}I-Iomazenil (IMP) and ^{123}I-Iofupane (DaTscanTM) are radiopharmaceuticals used in SPECT/CT in clinical routine [1, 2].

It facilitates the reconstruction of data across all required planes, such as axial, sagittal, and coronal, while greatly enhancing localization and contrast resolution in comparison with traditional planar imaging. Hybrid SPECT/CT imaging provides both anatomical information and higher resolution images with attenuation correction.

3. PET and PET/CT imaging

FDG is the most common tracer applied in PET neuroimaging to image cerebral glucose metabolism, thus providing more information on the etiopathogenesis of different neurological diseases. The radiotracers used in PET imaging for brain tumors

Blood-Brain-Barrier Agents	Cerebral Perfusion Agents	Cerebral Receptor-Binding Agents
Tc-99 m pertechnetate	I-123 N-isopropyl-p-iodoamphetamine (IMP)	I-123 ioflupane (DaTSCAN®)
Tc-99 m Diethylene-triaminepentaacetic acid (^{99m}Tc-DTPA)	Tc-99 m Hexamethylpropyleneamine Oxime (^{99m}Tc-HMPAO)	I-123 iodobenzamide (IBZM)
Thallium Chloride (^{201}TlCl)	Tc-99 m ethylene dicysteine (^{99m}Tc-ECD)	I-123 iomazenil (IMP)
Gallium-67 (^{67}Ga) Citrate	Thallium-201 diethyldithiocarbamate (^{201}TI-DDC)	Tc-99 m TRODAT-1
Tc-99 m Methoxyisobutilizonitrile (^{99m}Tc-MIBI)	Xenon-133 (^{133}Xe)	I-123-beta-carbomethoxy-3 beta-(4-iodophenyltropane) (CIT)
	Radiolabeled microsphere and macroaggregated albumin (MAA)	I-123 Fluoropropyl (FP)CIT
		I-123 Epidepride

Table 1.
SPECT radiopharmaceuticals for brain imaging.

Glucose metabolism	^{18}F-fluoro-deoxy-glucose (FDG)
Aminoacid metabolism, protein synthesis	^{18}F-fluoro-ethyl-l-tyrosine (FET)
	^{11}C-methionine (MET)
	^{18}F-Fluciclovine
	^{18}F-Fluorodopa (DOPA)
Amyloid imaging	^{18}F-Florbetapir (Amyvid®)
	^{18}F-Flutemetamol (Vizamyl®)
	^{18}F-Florbetaben (Neuraceq®)
	^{11}C-labeled Pittsburgh compound-B (^{11}C-PiB)
Thymidine metabolism, proliferation rate	^{18}F-Fluorothymidine (FLT)
	4′-methyl-^{11}C-thiothymidine(^{11}C-DST)
Oxygen metabolism	^{18}F-Fluoromisonidazole (FMISO)
Membrane biosynthesis, cell membrane	^{18}F-Fluorocholine
Tau imaging	^{18}F-AV1451 (also known as flortaucipir or T807)
Dopamine receptor imaging	^{124}I-epidepride
	^{18}F-fallypride
	^{11}C-raclopride (RAC)
	^{18}F-desmethoxyfallypride (DMFP)

Table 2.
PET radiopharmaceuticals for brain imaging.

can be categorized as agents targeting glucose metabolism, amino acid metabolism, cell proliferation, hypoxia, and other receptors (**Table 2**) [2]. FDG PET is a powerful diagnostic modality for early diagnosis and differential diagnosis of dementia disorders, evaluation of brain tumors, and detection of epileptic foci [2].

Amyloid and ^{18}F-flortaucipir PET are worthwhile imaging modalities that provide evidence of Alzheimer's pathophysiology and will be increasingly used in combination with ^{18}F-FDG PET images to further improve the diagnostic assessment of cognitive impairment and dementia [3].

4. Neurodegenerative disorders

Neurodegenerative disorders are chronic and progressive conditions characterized by the gradual loss of structure and function due to the accumulation of various abnormal protein aggregates in neurons, glial cells, and extracellular compartments in the central nervous system (CNS) and in peripheral organs [4]. The disorders differ according to the involvement of functional systems and are associated with a wide range of clinical presentations. They can be categorized according to the clinical features (e.g., dementia, parkinsonism, or motor neuron disease), anatomical regions affected by neurodegeneration (e.g., frontotemporal degenerations or extrapyramidal disorders), and underlying molecular abnormality.

4.1 Dementia-related neurodegenerative disorders

Dementia is an impairment of various cognitive functions, such as memory, language, and executive function, characterized by progressively worsening dysfunction beyond the expected range of normal aging [5]. Furthermore, advanced age is a major risk factor for dementia, and its prevalence is predicted to increase in the future as the average age of the population increases [6]. Therefore, early detection and classification of dementia has become an increasingly important topic.

Dementia is mostly caused by primary neurodegenerative disorders, which are defined by progressive, cumulative damage to neuronal structure, and interconnections. The most common diseases causing dementia are AD, followed by vascular dementia, DLB, and FTD, respectively [7, 8]. Additionally, rare neurodegenerative diseases such as an atypical Parkinson's syndrome known as progressive supranuclear palsy (PSP), posterior cortical atrophy (PCA), corticobasal degeneration, and multisystem atrophy (MSA) may also cause dementia. Thus, a timely and accurate diagnosis of these dementia-causing diseases is valuable to provide appropriate pharmacological treatment as well as to facilitate early non-pharmacological interventions, diminish healthcare costs, and provide prognostic information for the expected clinical course. However, there are diagnostic challenges due to the insidious onset of dementia and the significant symptomatic and clinical manifestations overlap between these diseases. The assessment and diagnostic process can be further complicated by other comorbidities such as depression, hypothyroidism, or cognitive impairment resulting from medications such as anticholinergics or benzodiazepines/barbiturates. Clinically, dementia syndromes can be diagnosed by exclusion combining medical history, physical examination, neuropsychological tests, laboratory evaluation, and neuroimaging modalities such as conventional anatomic imaging (CT and MRI) and hybrid imaging (fMRI, PET/CT, and PET/MRI).

FDG PET usually demonstrates similar metabolic activity in the cerebral cortex, caudate, and thalamus [9]. The pattern of glucose metabolism of the brain alters with normal aging, including reduced glucose uptake observed in the anterior and middle cingulate gyri and regions of the superior medial prefrontal cortex [10]. Some parts of the parietal and superior temporal poles are among other areas that may show decreased FDG uptake with normal aging. Generally, the metabolic activity of subcortical structures is not altered [10]. The most typical patterns of brain metabolic changes for neurodegenerative diseases are summarized in **Table 3**.

4.2 Alzheimer's disease

Alzheimer's disease (AD) is the most common neurodegenerative disorder associated with dementia. The onset of AD, a stereotypic dementia, is insidious and characterized by progressive episodic memory impairment with visuospatial or other cognitive dysfunction, followed by impairment in daily functioning. There is a wide spectrum of clinical manifestations ranging from mild cognitive impairment (MCI) to severe dementia. The severity of the disease is associated with the degree of neurodegeneration and pathological protein accumulation [11, 12].

Brain Regions	**Disorders**				
	AD	**DLB**	**FTD**	**PCA**	**Corticobasal Degeneration**
Temporoparietal cortex	✓	✓	Possible	✓[1]	✓[2]
Frontal lobe	*	***	✓	Preserved	✓[2]
Precuneus	✓	✓	Preserved	✓[1]	✓[2]
Anterior Temporal lobe	Relatively preserved	Variable	✓	Preserved	Preserved
Posterior cingulate gyrus	✓	Island sign	Possible	✓[1]	✓[2]
Anterior cingulate gyrus	Preserved	Variable	✓	Preserved	✓
Visual cortex	Preserved	✓	Preserved	Preserved	Preserved
Occipital lobe	**	✓	Preserved	✓	Preserved
Primary sensorimotor cortex	Preserved	Preserved	Variable to preserved	Preserved	✓[2]
Basal ganglia	Preserved	✓ (caudate)	Variable to preserved	Preserved	✓[2]

Abbreviations: AD, Alzheimer's disease; FTD, frontotemporal dementia (behavioral variant); DLB, dementia with Lewy bodies; PCA, posterior cortical atrophy. **Frontal hypometabolism may present in more advanced stages of AD or in the frontal variant of AD (dorsolateral and orbitofrontal cortex).*
***Hypometabolism in the occipital lobe may present in the posterior variant of AD (associative and primary visual cortex).*
****Frontal hypometabolism may present in more with advanced DLB.*
[1]*Hypometabolism in temporoparietal cortex, precuneus, and posterior cingulate gyrus may be present in PCA but are usually more asymmetric than in DLB.*
[2]*In corticobasal syndrome, normal or asymmetrically decreased FDG uptake can occur.*

Table 3.
Brain FDG PET Patterns of Hypometabolism in Dementia-Related Neurodegenerative Diseases.

The amyloid-β plaques, pathologic tau deposition, and neurodegeneration (A/T/N) staging system have been recommended for the evaluation of patients at risk of AD [13]. Among neuroimaging modalities, amyloid and tau PET are important topographic biomarkers of amyloid and tau deposition. Neurodegeneration consists of both reduced metabolic neuronal function evaluated by FDG PET and structural changes such as volume loss demonstrated by MRI.

FDG PET, a marker of neurodegeneration and progression, is one of the most widely used imaging modalities for the evaluation of AD with a variety of indications as follows:

1. In predicting the progression from MCI to AD.

2. Early diagnosis of suspected AD and differential diagnosis from other causes of dementia such as dementia with Lewy bodies (DLB), frontotemporal degeneration (FTD), and vascular dementia (VD).

3. Differential diagnosis of AD variants with atypical clinical presentation [14].

Mild cognitive impairment (MCI) is a clinical transitional condition between normal aging and dementia, characterized by a decline in neurocognitive functioning that does not affect activities of daily living according to the patient's age and educational status. Predicting the prognosis of MCI patients is difficult because they can develop into various types of dementia or remain stable and even return to normal [15]. However, FDG PET scan has been used to predict the prognosis of MCI [8]. The pattern of hypometabolism in the posterior cingulate and posterior temporoparietal areas has an important role in predicting patients who may progress from MCI to AD [15, 16].

In typical AD, FDG PET scan revealed hypometabolism in the posterior cingulate gyrus, precuneus, and posterior temporal and parietal lobes, whereas metabolic activity was preserved in the primary sensorimotor and primary visual cortices, basal ganglia, thalamus, pons, and cerebellum (**Figure 1**). Hypometabolism in the frontal lobes may be present in more advanced stages of AD or the frontal variant of AD [17]. This metabolic pattern on FDG PET has been shown to have high sensitivity and specificity (>90% for both) for distinguishing AD from healthy elderly controls. The specificity of FDG PET for discrimination between AD and other types of dementia (including MCI) is around 78% [18, 19].

Some AD cases exhibit unusual clinical features, primarily characterized by dominant symptoms related to visuospatial abilities, language, or behavioral/executive dysfunction, which are categorized as visual variant or posterior cortical atrophy (PCA), logopenic variant primary progressive aphasia (lvPPA), and frontal variant AD (fvAD) of the disease. These variants are usually present at an earlier age than typical amnestic AD, and the memory functions tend to be relatively intact [8, 17].

Posterior cortical atrophy (PCA) is a posterior or visual variant of AD with marked atrophy of parietooccipital cortical areas dominated by symptoms such as visual-perceptual deficits, extremity apraxia or ignorance, and reduced ability to interpret, locate, and identify objects, symbols, words, and faces [20]. PCA can be differentiated from typical AD by asymmetric hypometabolism in the lateral occipital cortices (visual association cortex) [7, 21]. Although PCA and DLB may exhibit similar patterns of hypometabolism, PCA tends to show more asymmetric and larger hypometabolism in the lateral occipital cortex and parietal cortex than DLB (**Figure 2**) [12, 21, 22].

As a PPA variant most often accompanied by AD pathology, the lvPPA is characterized by anomia, difficulty in repeating complex sentences, and phonological errors,

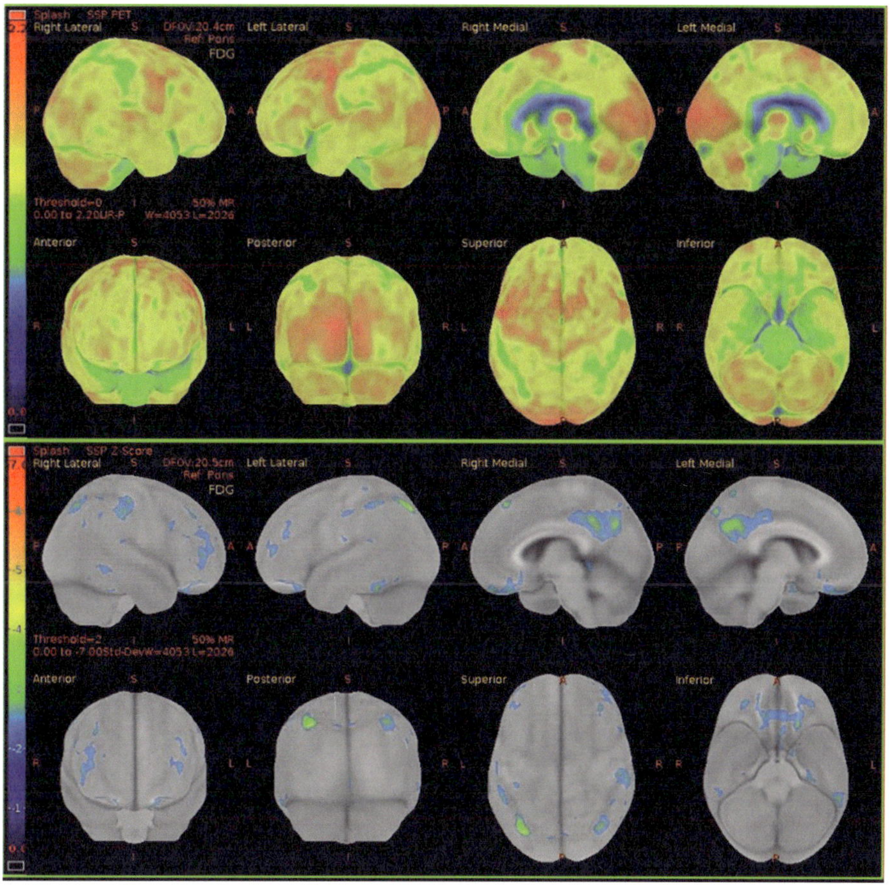

Figure 1.
A 67-year-old female patient had complaints of increasing forgetfulness and inability to perform daily tasks for 3 years. On visual assessment, hypometabolism has been observed in bilateral precuneus, and bilateral parietal lobe inferior in the posterior cingulate and was evaluated as early-stage AD (CortexID, GE Healthcare).

affecting language abilities [23]. The right medial temporal and posterior cingulate gyrus, typically the temporal lobe and the left supramarginal gyrus, show patterns of hypometabolism that may be associated with language impairments (**Figure 3**) [24, 25]. FDG PET has a diagnostic role in distinguishing lvPPA from other types of PPA [26].

The clinical presentation of the frontal variant of AD, which resembles the behavioral variant of frontotemporal dementia (bvFTD), is characterized by progressive apathy or behavioral disinhibition and stereotypic executive dysfunction. Therefore, combining FDG PET and amyloid PET scans may contribute to the differential diagnosis of fvAD from bvFTD [27]. Hypometabolism in medial-frontal and orbitofrontal areas has been shown in FvAH [17].

The characteristic pattern of hypometabolism expected in AD pathology may be abnormal on FDG PET, in which case amyloid PET may help clarify the diagnosis. Studies comparing the results of PET and autopsy evaluating the success of amyloid PET with ^{18}F-labeled radiotracer in detecting positive amyloid plaques in elderly individuals found sensitivity between 82 and 98% and specificity between 80 and 95% [28, 29]. The amyloid radiotracers ^{11}C-Pittsburgh compound B (^{11}C-PIB) and ^{18}F-florbetapir,

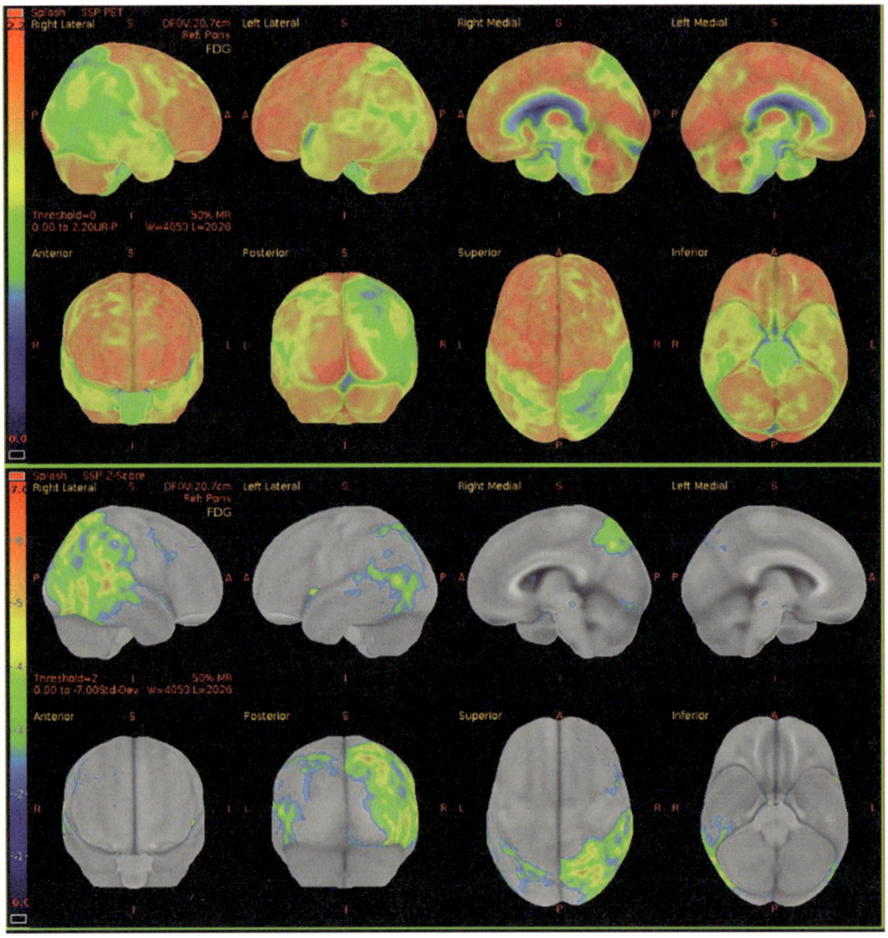

Figure 2.
A 61-year-old female patient underwent brain FDG PET examination because of forgetfulness, visual and functional impairment for 2 years. On visual evaluation, hypometabolism has been found in the parietal, temporal and occipital lobes, more prominent on the right and was compatible with posterior cortical atrophy (PCA) (CortexID, GE Healthcare).

^{18}F-florbetaben, and ^{18}F-flutemetamol (^{18}F-FMM) have specific characteristics and differences in procedural standards and acceptable interpretation methods.

Normal amyloid PET scans have a clear white-gray matter distinction. On the PET scans, in patients with significant Aß deposition, the distinction between the white and gray matter junction is blurred, depending on the amount of radiotracer uptake observed in the gray matter [30]. Activity uptake in gray and white matter tends to be symmetrical. The posterior cingulate cortex, precuneus, parietal, lateral temporal, and frontal lobes have radiotracer uptake, while the sensorimotor cortex and visual cortices are comparatively preserved. Also, the presence of cerebral atrophy and widening of the sulci may lead to a misleading perception of normal white matter uptake that appears dendritic pattern. Conscientious correlation with anatomical imaging can help overcome these pitfalls.

Amyloid PET scan is positive in the typical presentation and atypical variants of AD. A negative amyloid PET rules out the diagnosis of AD, but the amyloid PET with a positive pattern is not pathognomonic for AD. The deposition of amyloid is

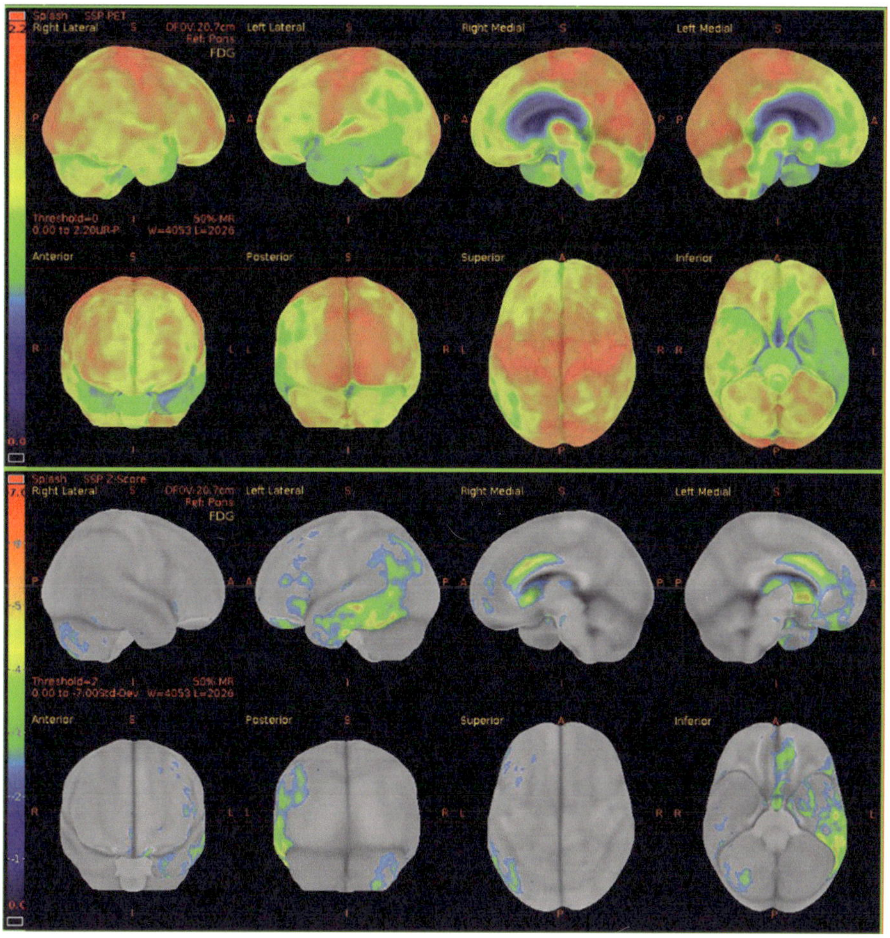

Figure 3.
A 73-year-old female with complaints of anomia, word repetition and reading impairment for 1 year underwent FDG PET. Hypometabolism was observed in the prefrontal lateral section, temporal and parietal lobes in the left cerebral hemisphere and logopenic variant primary progressive aphasia was diagnosed when evaluated with clinical findings (CortexID, GE Healthcare).

associated with normal aging, and amyloid positivity can be seen even in cognitively normal individuals, some non-AD dementias, such as DLB and cerebral amyloid angiopathy [31]. Therefore, it is necessary to evaluate the patient's symptoms more comprehensively with other biomarkers.

Currently, ^{18}F-flortaucipir (AV-1451) is the only US FDA-approved tau radiotracer with affinity for the helical filament tau. There is other non-AD neurodegenerative tauopathies characterized by tau protein accumulation such as Pick disease, DLB, sporadic corticobasal degeneration, and progressive supranuclear palsy. It is only indicated to demonstrate tau burden in cognitively impaired patients being evaluated for AD.

Particularly abnormal ^{18}F-flortaucipir uptake in the posterolateral temporal quadrant, parietal lobe/precuneus, or occipital lobes may be considered positive for diffusely distributed tau pathology. The radiotracer uptake in the medial or anterolateral temporal lobes, frontal lobes, or deep gray nuclei and white matter is considered non-specific off-target and a negative scan [3]. Tau protein deposition increases with the progression of AD and can be used to determine disease severity and staging [32].

4.3 Dementia with Lewy body

Dementia with Lewy body (DLB), the second leading neurodegenerative disease in people over 65 years of age, is characterized by fluctuating cognition, slow-onset recurrent visual hallucinations, rapid eye movement sleep behavior disorder, and spontaneous parkinsonism [33]. In the early stages of DLB, memory functions are preserved compared to AD. The underlying pathology in DLB is characterized by Lewy bodies formed by the accumulation of abnormally folded intracellular alpha-synuclein protein in cortical, subcortical, and some brainstem neurons [34]. Intact Lewy bodies eventually lead to impaired axonal transport, synaptic dysfunction, and cell death.

Parkinson's disease dementia (PDD) and DLB have the same clinical spectrum and are differentiated according to the time of onset of symptoms. In DLB, cognitive symptoms and then motor manifestations have been observed. The diagnosis of probable DLB is usually based on the clinical findings described above. DLB and PDD have less prominent and nonspecific findings in anatomical imaging modalities compared to AD and FTD. Compared with AD, the medial temporal lobe is preserved from atrophy in DLB and PDD [35].

In DLD and PDD, there is hypometabolism in the frontal, parietal, and medial occipital lobe, including the primary visual cortex, but the medial temporal-hippocampal region is relatively spared (**Figure 4**). The posterior cingulate island sign (CIS), which indicates a relatively preserved metabolism in the posterior cingulate gyrus compared to the precuneus, is a DLB-specific finding and is important in the differential diagnosis of AD and PDD [36].

DAT imaging with SPECT using radiotracer ^{123}I-Ioflupane (DaTscanTM) is an important imaging modality for the assessment of vivo dopaminergic function. In DLB and Parkinson's disease (PD), loss of dopaminergic neurons extending from the substantia nigra to the striatum and nigrostriatal degeneration, and decreased radiotracer uptake in the striatum is observed on DAT SPECT [37]. Therefore, the decrease in radiotracer uptake in the striatum occurs posterior to the putamen, and

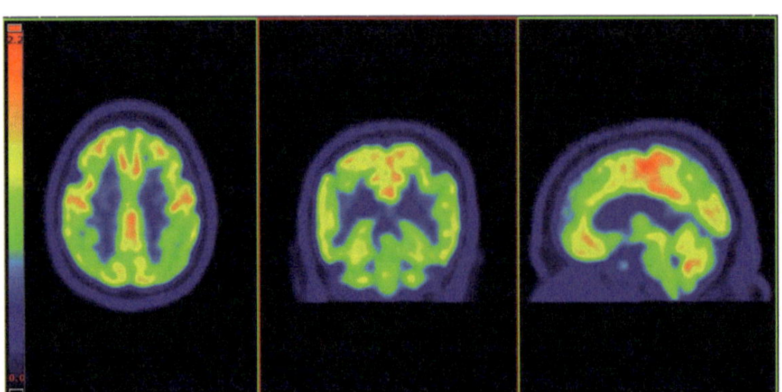

Figure 4.
A 70-year-old man with complaints of visual hallucinations, slowing of left dominant movements and forgetfulness underwent FDG PET. Hypometabolism was observed in bilateral parietal lobes, bilateral precuneus, bilateral occipital lateral and lower intensity primary visual cortices, more prominent on the left, and dementia with Lewy Body (DLB) was diagnosed.

since the caudate head is preserved, the comma appearance normally observed in the striatum disappears and turns into a dot shape. While it cannot discriminate between PD and DLB, it has an important role in differentiating between DLB and AD due to the preservation of radioactivity uptake in the striatum in AD [38].

^{123}I-MIBG cardiac scintigraphy is utilized to evaluate cardiac postganglionic sympathetic degeneration, a general feature in neurodegenerative diseases with Lewy bodies pathology. DLB characteristically shows a decrease in cardiac MIBG uptake. However, false positive results may be obtained in the presence of diabetes mellitus or heart disease [39].

4.4 Frontotemporal dementia

Frontotemporal dementia (FTD) is a spectrum of syndromes characterized by progressive deterioration in behavior, language, and cognitive functions pathologically associated with selective degeneration in the cortical and subcortical frontal and temporal lobes. It is the third most common cause of dementia in those over 65 years of age and the most common cause of early-onset dementia. In FTD, patients frequently present with personality and behavioral changes and decreased speaking and physical skills. However, FTD is used as a hypernym term referring to three main variants: behavioral variant frontotemporal dementia (bvFTD), semantic variant primary progressive aphasia (svPPA), and nonfluent/grammatical variant PPA (nfvPPA) [40]. These subtypes have different clinical symptoms and different metabolic markers.

The classical FTD is mainly defined by hypometabolism in the frontal and anterior temporal lobes and the involvement of the anterior cingulate gyrus [7]. The bvFTD, also known as frontal variant FTD, is the most common FTD clinically presenting with behavioral disinhibition, loss of empathy, and hyperorality. FDG PET reveals asymmetric, bilateral hypometabolism in the frontal lobes, anterior cingulate gyrus, and anterior temporal lobes. The hypometabolism areas are generally consistent in localization with atrophy patterns and have larger effect sizes [41].

Primary progressive aphasia (PPA) is characterized by language impairment occurring in the relative absence of cognitive impairment, behavioral impairment, or motor symptoms. The main PPAs are non-fluent, semantic, and logopenic; the first two are categorized as FTD subtypes while the last is an AD subtype. The main features of the nfvPPA include agrammatism, consisting of a nonsensical, halting, and disorganized speech pattern. The hypometabolism in the left ventrolateral prefrontal cortex (PFC), and supplementary motor area is observed on FDG PET [42]. svFTD is clinically described by the main features of impaired confrontational naming and single-word comprehension. In the svFTD, FDG PET may show hypometabolism in the anterior temporal lobe with more prominence in the left [43].

4.5 Vascular dementia and other conditions

Vascular dementia (VD) is the most common cause of dementia among non-neurodegenerative diseases, and other central nervous system diseases such as alcohol-related dementia, chronic traumatic encephalopathy, normal pressure hydrocephalus, and chronic subdural hematoma are less common etiologies [12].

Depression is the most common cause of pseudodementia. The prevalence of dementia and depression increases with aging. Symptoms of pseudodementia are associated with depression, but depression in the elderly is considered a risk factor for dementia. Clinically, it is not easy to distinguish between these two conditions. Moreover, a normal or preserved pattern of cerebral uptake on FDG PET may help distinguish reversible pseudodementia due to depression from primary neurodegenerative disorder [44, 45].

Alcohol-induced cognitive impairment and Wernicke's encephalopathy are potentially reversible cognitive disorders. Alcohol abstinence typically shows amelioration of cognition-related clinical functions. FDG PET has demonstrated the most prominent hypometabolic changes in the medial and lateral frontal cortex as well as in the anterior cingulate gyrus [46].

In genetically inherited Huntington's disease (HD), which also causes slowly progressive movement and behavioral disorders, and dementia, marked hypometabolism, especially in the caudate nucleus and putamen, can be observed in the early stages [47].

5. Movement disorders

Movement disorders can be roughly divided into hypokinetic (lack of movement) and hyperkinetic (abnormal unintentional movements). The clinical picture that occurs in these diseases is called parkinsonism because Parkinson's disease (PD) is the prototype and most common cause of hypokinetic movement disorder. Other diseases in this group show similar clinical findings with PD and constitute the main area of interest in nuclear medicine.

Idiopathic PD is the second leading neurodegenerative disease after Alzheimer's disease. The main clinical symptoms of parkinsonism are resting tremors, rigidity, bradykinesia, and postural instability, as well as dementia, cognitive impairment, and cranial nerve dysfunction. Besides, these findings are also present in multi-system atrophy (MSA), progressive supranuclear palsy (PSP), corticobasal degeneration (CBD), and dementia with Lewy bodies (LCD), which are called Parkinson plus syndromes (PPS), also known as atypical parkinsonism [48]. However, it is not easy to clinically differentiate the PPS with neurodegenerative features from PD, especially in the early period [49]. Furthermore, essential tremor (ET) which does not cause loss of dopaminergic neurons and other secondary causes of parkinsonism (due to drug use, cerebrovascular event, trauma, or infection) should be clinically distinguished from PD. As all these diseases have different prognoses and treatments, it is important to make a correct differential diagnosis [48]. Presynaptic or postsynaptic imaging of the dopaminergic system by nuclear medicine imaging methods has an important role in the differential diagnosis of parkinsonism. Thus, they are used in parkinsonism to determine striatal dopamine deficiency and provide early dopamine replacement therapy or to demonstrate the integrity of the dopaminergic system and avoid unnecessary dopamine replacement therapy [50].

5.1 Presynaptic dopaminergic imaging

Brain SPECT imaging with ^{123}I-Ioflupane (DaTscanTM) was performed in the follow-up of patients with a clinically uncertain diagnosis, especially in those with a suspected essential tremor, drug-induced parkinsonism, or vascular parkinsonism [51]. It shows high sensitivity in the differential diagnosis of essential tremor [50]. In the axial section of SPECT, normal striatal nuclei can be clearly distinguished from the surrounding tissue in a comma shape. PD is excluded in negative scans detecting a bilateral comma shape. In PD, presynaptic dopaminergic loss usually starts asymmetrically in the posterior putamen; as the disease progresses, this decrease extends to the anterior putamen and caudate nucleus and appears bilaterally [52]. Nevertheless, it is an insufficient imaging method in the differential diagnosis of PD from parkinsonism syndromes with neurodegenerative causes due to their similar findings.

^{18}F-Fluorodopa (DOPA) is a PET radiopharmaceutical used to assess presynaptic dopaminergic integrity, dopamine metabolism by dopa-decarboxylase, dopamine storage capacity, and nigrostriatal dopaminergic deficit. It effectively differentiates normal individuals from Parkinson's patients. Still, it is less reliable in differentiating PD from PPS such as MSA and PSP and in distinguishing ex novo PD from advanced PD [53, 54].

5.2 Postsynaptic dopaminergic imaging

These modalities are often used to differentiate PD from MSA and PSP. Dopamine D2 receptor SPECT and PET studies using commercially accessible radiopharmaceuticals ^{123}I-Iodobenzamide (IBZM) and ^{123}I-epidepride, as well as ^{11}C-raclopride, ^{18}F-fallypride, and ^{18}F-desmethoxyfallypride (DMFP) [55]. They show normal or increased radiopharmaceutical uptake in the basal ganglia in PD, whereas this uptake is decreased in other PPS such as MSA and PSP. Therefore, with high diagnostic accuracy, they can distinguish PD from other parkinsonism syndromes [55–57].

5.3 ^{18}F-FDG PET imaging

Brain FDG PET imaging is mainly performed for the differential diagnosis of PD and PPS [58]. According to the glucose metabolism pattern associated with PD, which is known as the Parkinson's disease-related pattern (PDRP), hypometabolism is observed in premotor, supplementary motor, and parietal cortical regions; hypermetabolism is observed in bilateral basal ganglia, thalamus, pons, and cerebellum, being prominent in dorsolateral putamen [59]. Based on brain FDG PET imaging findings, diagnostic classification overlaps with the definitive clinical diagnosis by 90% and neurodegenerative causes of parkinsonism (PD, MSA, PSP, and LCD) can be differentiated by 90% [60]. The severity and extent of abnormal findings on brain FDG PET imaging in parkinsonism syndromes are usually related to clinical findings [48, 61, 62].

Multi-system atrophy (MSA) is a rare, sporadic, and progressive neurodegenerative disease that occurs between 50 and 60 years of age. It is characterized by autonomic dysfunction such as cerebellar ataxia, urinary dysfunction, and orthostatic hypotension as well as parkinsonism findings [63]. In MSA, a hypometabolic uptake pattern is observed in the basal ganglia and cerebellum, and this difference in uptake pattern provides a differential diagnosis between MSA and PD [48, 59]. Hypometabolism in the cerebellum is a diagnostic finding that helps the differential diagnosis of MSA because it is not observed in other neurodegenerative diseases included in the differential diagnosis of parkinsonism. Similarly, bilateral basal ganglia involvement in MSA is a supportive finding regarding differential diagnosis with CBD in which asymmetric basal ganglia involvement is detected [64].

Progressive supranuclear palsy (PSP) is a neurodegenerative disorder characterized by tau protein accumulation in neurons and glial cells, particularly in the brain stem, basal ganglia, and frontal cortex, with clinical manifestations of parkinsonism and dementia. Patients have impaired eye movements (supranuclear gaze palsy; particularly difficulty with downward gaze), pseudobulbar palsy, and axial dystonia. FDG PET demonstrates hypometabolism in the prefrontal cortex, frontal eye fields, medial thalamus, caudate nuclei, and upper brain stem [61, 65].

Corticobasal degeneration (CBD) is a rare neurodegenerative disease with a typically asymmetric onset, and patients have some clinical manifestations such as akinetic-rigid syndrome, dystonia, myoclonus, apraxia, cortical sensory loss, dysarthria, eye movement disturbance, and foreign hand syndrome. It is characterized by hypometabolism in the bilateral caudate and thalamic nucleus, parietal lobe, middle frontal, and cingulate gyrus, more prominent in the cerebral hemisphere contralateral to the most affected side of the body [59, 61].

5.4 ^{123}I-MIBG cardiac scintigraphy

Myocardial scintigraphy with ^{123}I-metaiodobenzylguanidine (MIBG) is used to evaluate postganglionic presynaptic cardiac sympathetic nerve endings in cardiac diseases such as congestive heart failure, ischemic heart disease, and cardiomyopathy. Cardiac MIBG uptake was reduced in patients with Lewy body diseases such as PD and DLB, but not in patients with MSA and PSP patients [66]. Thus, it was useful for differentiating PD from other parkinsonism and DLB from AD. However, normal cardiac MIBG does not rule out the diagnosis of PD in patients with suspected Parkinson's syndrome [67].

6. Epilepsy

Epilepsy is an important chronic neurological disease characterized by sudden and recurrent seizures, resulting from abnormal and excessive electrical discharge in cortical neurons. Optimal seizure control is not achieved in approximately one-third of the cases treated with antiepileptic therapy, leading to serious morbidity and mortality. The epileptic foci can be surgically removed in appropriate patient groups to reduce the number and prevalence of epileptic seizures, improve the patient's quality of life, and reduce drug-related side effects.

Various functional imaging modalities are used for lateralization and epileptogenic foci detection (temporal and extratemporal epilepsy) before surgical intervention. Among nuclear medicine imaging modalities, brain SPECT with Tc-99 m hexamethyl propylenamine oxime (HMPAO) or ethylene dicysteine (ECD) or brain FDG PET are frequently used for this purpose. Imaging studies are defined as ictal (at the time of seizure), interictal (during the seizure-free period), or postictal (immediately after the seizure) according to the timing of the injection. ^{18}F-Flumazenil (FMZ) also shows the seizure zone but is localized in a more limited area than FDG [68].

In ictal SPECT, the radiopharmaceutical injection is performed intravenously at the onset or during a seizure under EEG monitoring. The expected image pattern is hyperperfusion in the epileptogenic zone. The hyperperfusion in the same-sided basal ganglia, thalamus, and motor cortex or hypoperfusion in the contralateral cerebellar hemisphere due to diaschisis related to the supratentorial seizure foci are additional important findings for lateralization of the epileptogenic zone. Ictal SPECT performed under optimal conditions is 90% in temporal lobe epilepsies (TLE) and 70–83% in extratemporal lobe epilepsies (ETLE) in identifying the epileptogenic focus [69]. Interictal SPECT is performed in the inter-seizure period. The image pattern is hypoperfusion or normal perfusion in the epileptogenic focus. The sensitivity of interictal SPECT is less than that of ictal SPECT [69]. Additionally, Subtraction Ictal SPECT Co-registered to MRI (SISCOM) is a high-resolution imaging technique that enables the detection of epileptic focus with high sensitivity and specificity by comparing ictal and interictal perfusion images [70].

PET provides valuable information for the detection of epileptogenic focus in cases with no findings on EEG and MRI. However, FDG PET is not appropriate for assessing short-term neuronal changes because it requires approximately 30–60 minutes after injection for transport and accumulation in the brain parenchyma. In interictal FDG PET, hypometabolism in the epileptogenic zone is the characteristic image pattern. The sensitivity of FDG PET imaging in demonstrating the epileptogenic region has been reported to be 90–95% in TLE and 42–92% in ETLE. Although it has a low sensitivity in ETLE, clinical evaluation may be useful considering that MRI findings are normal in this patient population [71].

The location and number of epileptogenic foci are crucial factors influencing treatment management of drug-resistant epilepsy (DRE) such as surgery or neuromodulatory interventions. Generally, the treatment response is defined as seizure reduction >50% of baseline. FDG PET can provide lateralizing and localizing information in patients with DRE undergoing presurgical evaluation. Patients with unsafe lesion location, unacceptably high risk of neurological deficit after surgery, multifocal or poorly localized epilepsy foci, or continued seizures following a previous resection are generally not suitable for surgery and may benefit from neuromodulation interventions.

PET/MRI is a promising hybrid imaging modality that improves epilepsy evaluation by combining metabolic and structural imaging. Recent studies suggest that PET/MRI fusion imaging improves the sensitivity and specificity of detecting epileptogenic foci, especially in cases with subtle cortical dysplasia or mesial temporal sclerosis [72].

7. Brain death scintigraphy

Brain death is the irreversible cessation of all brain functions, including brain stem functions. Intracranial blood flow has ceased. Nowadays, with increasing developments in organ transplantation, the diagnosis of brain death is becoming gradually more important for the identification of transplant donors. Brain scintigraphy is used to confirm the diagnosis of brain death by assessing cerebral blood flow to show that all functions of the cerebrum and brainstem have irreversibly ceased. Also, it is a cost-effective, easily performed, and non-invasive technique. It is particularly helpful when clinical examinations are inconclusive due to interfering factors such as drug intoxication, metabolic disorders or severe cranial trauma because it is not affected by drug intoxication and hypothermia.

The method provides a precise and objective assessment of brain function by detecting the absence of cerebral perfusion. Brain-specific (hydrophobic) radiopharmaceuticals commonly used in the scintigraphy include ^{99m}Tc-ECD, ^{99m}Tc-HMPAO, which readily cross the blood–brain barrier and accumulate in brain. Alternatively, non-specific brain (hydrophilic) perfusion agents such as ^{99m}Tc-pertechnetate (with perchlorate blockade), ^{99m}Tc-diethylene-triamine-pentaacetate (DTPA), and ^{99m}Tc-glucoheptonate can be used to evaluate cerebral blood flow dynamics [73].

The procedure consists of dynamic imaging in the anterior projection immediately after radiotracer injection, followed by delayed static images and sometimes SPECT/CT. Absence of flow and perfusion in the middle cerebral artery, anterior cerebral artery, and posterior cerebral artery on brain scan confirms brain death. In late static imaging, brain activity is absent, "hollow skull phenomenon" in brain death cases [74]. Additionally, the "hot nose" sign associated with a relative increase in external carotid artery flow may be observed, which may manifest as a markedly increased radiopharmaceutical uptake in the nasal region of the patient [75].

Brain death scintigraphy offers several advantages over other diagnostic modalities. Contrast-enhanced cerebral angiography, digital-subtraction angiography (DSA), and contrast-enhanced computed tomography (CT) are more expensive procedures, and additionally, contrast agents are administered. These agents can be toxic to the kidney and should be considered if the patient is a donor candidate for kidney transplantation. In addition, in brain death, intracranial pressure increases because of brain oedema, necrosis, and autolysis, and these changes may cause false negatives on CT or MRI. Nevertheless, brain scintigraphy is a reliable imaging modality with low false-positive results when performed correctly. It can also be repeated as needed without any concern about radiation exposure or impairment of kidney function.

8. Neuro-oncology

SPECT and SPECT/CT are used in the diagnosis of brain tumors, especially in the diagnosis of recurrent gliomas and lymphomas. The most important feature of SPECT radiopharmaceuticals is that they cross the blood–brain barrier (BBB) and localize in brain tissue such as ^{99m}Tc-ECD, ^{99m}Tc-HMPAO, demonstrating brain perfusion. Brain perfusion SPECT can be used to determine the type of malignancy/indeterminate tumors and to differentiate intracranial lymphomas from toxoplasmosis. Brain tumors most commonly present with increased radiotracer uptake compared to normal parenchyma [76]. Besides, brain tumors imaging with thallium-201 (201Tl) reflects more accurately live tumor burden than radionuclide studies with CT, MRI or other single-photon emitting compounds [77]. SPECT images have lower spatial resolution than PET images. Therefore, these tracers are currently used in clinical practice to investigate brain tumors.

PET scans are indicated in patients with brain tumors for initial staging, evaluation of residual mass after surgery, re-staging, differential diagnosis from suspected recurrence or radiation necrosis, and evaluation of response to treatment. They are frequently used in the differential diagnosis between tumor recurrence and radiation injury. For assessing brain tumors, a variety of conventional and novel radiotracers have been developed [78].

FDG PET can predict tumor grading in vivo better than other techniques because generally higher metabolic activity indicates higher tumor grade. Amino acid radiotracers exhibit a high sensitivity to their movement across the blood-brain barrier and, to a limited extent, to the protein synthesis. Amino acid radiotracers [^{11}C-methionine, and ^{18}F-Fluorodopa (FDOPA),^{18}F-fluorothymidine (FLT)] are particularly effective in distinguishing between tumor recurrence and radiation-induced necrosis. Various tracers have been developed to investigate distinct biochemical activities, such as hypoxia (^{18}F-fluoromisonidazole), DNA replication (^{18}F-fluorothymidine), and membrane proliferation (^{11}C-choline or ^{18}F-fluorocholine) [78].

Locoregional radioimmunotherapy (RIT) targeting brain tumors with monoclonal antibodies (MoAb) conjugated with high-energy β-emitters (^{131}I, ^{90}Y, or ^{177}Lu) is proposed. Furthermore, tumor cells that do not express the antigen on their surface may be damaged by the "crossfire effect" [79].

9. Discussion and conclusion

In different neurological diseases, PET/CT and SPECT/CT hybrid imaging modalities can provide physiological and anatomical information from the central nervous system, helping clinicians to make reasonable and early diagnosis for prognosis and optimal patient management.

An important development in neuroimaging is the usage of hybrid PET/MRI systems that combine the soft tissue contrast of MRI with the functional and molecular imaging capabilities of PET. This integration provides more comprehensive information about neurological diseases and improves diagnostic accuracy.

Furthermore, the application of quantitative imaging biomarkers in nuclear medicine allows for more objective and reproducible assessments that can improve disease monitoring and treatment evaluation. Future research should focus on improving these technologies and integrating them into routine clinical practice to maximize their diagnostic and therapeutic potential. Collaboration between researchers, clinicians, and technology developers will be crucial in translating these innovations into practical applications that improve patient care and outcomes.

As functional neuroimaging has continued to develop, emerging trends are modeling their future impact. The image interpretation, pattern recognition, and the integration of artificial intelligence (AI) into neuroimaging workflows are improving diagnostic accuracy and efficiency through automated analysis and pattern recognition. Ultra-high-resolution imaging technologies improve diagnostic possibilities by enabling earlier detection of impairment in brain structure and function. Furthermore, the development of new radiopharmaceuticals is widening the range of molecular targets, improving disease characterization and treatment monitoring. These innovations collectively highlight the rapid development of functional neuroimaging and its growing impact on clinical practice and research.

Author details

Nur Aydinbelge Dizdar[1*] and Derya Cayir[1,2]

1 Department of Nuclear Medicine, Ankara Etlik City Hospital, Ankara, Turkiye

2 Department of Nuclear Medicine, University of Health Sciences, Ankara, Turkiye

*Address all correspondence to: fnuraydinbelge@gmail.com

References

[1] Saha GB, MacIntyre WJ, Go RT. Radiopharmaceuticals for brain imaging. Seminars in Nuclear Medicine. 1994;**24**(4):324-349

[2] Crișan G, Moldovean-Cioroianu NS, Timaru DG, Andrieș G, Căinap C, Chiș V. Radiopharmaceuticals for PET and SPECT Imaging: A Literature Review over the Last Decade. International Journal of Molecular Sciences. 30 Apr 2022;**23**(9):5023

[3] Burkett BJ, Johnson DR, Lowe VJ. Evaluation of neurodegenerative disorders with amyloid-β, tau, and dopaminergic PET imaging: Interpretation pitfalls. Journal of Nuclear Medicine. 2024;**65**(6):829-837

[4] Kovacs GG. Concepts and classification of neurodegenerative diseases. Handbook of Clinical Neurology. 2017;**145**:301-307

[5] Gallucci M, Limbucci N, Catalucci A, Caulo M. Neurodegenerative diseases. Radiologic Clinics of North America. 2008;**46**(4):799-817 vii

[6] Albanese E, Cataldi R, Guerche M, Nichols E, Prince M, Seeher K, et al. Global Status Report on the Public Health Response to Dementia. Geneva: World Health Organization; 2021

[7] Brown RK, Bohnen NI, Wong KK, Minoshima S, Frey KA. Brain PET in suspected dementia: Patterns of altered FDG metabolism. Radiographics. 2014;**34**(3):684-701

[8] Guillén EF, Rosales JJ, Lisei D, Grisanti F, Riverol M, Arbizu J. Current role of 18F-FDG-PET in the differential diagnosis of the main forms of dementia. Clinical and Translational Imaging. 2020;**8**(3):127-140

[9] Shivamurthy VK, Tahari AK, Marcus C, Subramaniam RM. Brain FDG PET and the diagnosis of dementia. AJR. American Journal of Roentgenology. 2015;**204**(1):W76-W85

[10] Kalpouzos G, Chételat G, Baron JC, Landeau B, Mevel K, Godeau C, et al. Voxel-based mapping of brain gray matter volume and glucose metabolism profiles in normal aging. Neurobiology of Aging. 2009;**30**(1):112-124

[11] Elahi FM, Miller BL. A clinicopathological approach to the diagnosis of dementia. Nature Reviews. Neurology. 2017;**13**(8):457-476

[12] Dave A, Hansen N, Downey R, Johnson C. FDG-PET imaging of dementia and neurodegenerative disease. Seminars in Ultrasound, CT, and MR. 2020;**41**(6):562-571

[13] Jack CR Jr, Bennett DA, Blennow K, Carrillo MC, Feldman HH, Frisoni GB, et al. A/T/N: An unbiased descriptive classification scheme for Alzheimer disease biomarkers. Neurology. 2016;**87**(5):539-547

[14] Guedj E, Varrone A, Boellaard R, Albert NL, Barthel H, van Berckel B, et al. EANM procedure guidelines for brain PET imaging using [(18)F]FDG, version 3. European Journal of Nuclear Medicine and Molecular Imaging. 2022;**49**(2):632-651

[15] Arbizu J, Festari C, Altomare D, Walker Z, Bouwman F, Rivolta J, et al. Clinical utility of FDG-PET for the clinical diagnosis in MCI. European Journal of Nuclear Medicine and Molecular Imaging. 2018;**45**(9):1497-1508

[16] Silverman DH, Small GW, Chang CY, Lu CS, Kung De Aburto MA, Chen W,

et al. Positron emission tomography in evaluation of dementia: Regional brain metabolism and long-term outcome. JAMA. 2001;**286**(17):2120-2127

[17] Sala A, Caprioglio C, Santangelo R, Vanoli EG, Iannaccone S, Magnani G, et al. Brain metabolic signatures across the Alzheimer's disease spectrum. European Journal of Nuclear Medicine and Molecular Imaging. 2020;**47**(2):256-269

[18] Bloudek LM, Spackman DE, Blankenburg M, Sullivan SD. Review and meta-analysis of biomarkers and diagnostic imaging in Alzheimer's disease. Journal of Alzheimer's Disease. 2011;**26**(4):627-645

[19] Khoury R, Ghossoub E. Diagnostic biomarkers of Alzheimer's disease: A state-of-the-art review. Biomarkers in Neuropsychiatry. 2019;**1**:100005

[20] Crutch SJ, Lehmann M, Schott JM, Rabinovici GD, Rossor MN, Fox NC. Posterior cortical atrophy. Lancet Neurology. 2012;**11**(2):170-178

[21] Whitwell JL, Graff-Radford J, Singh TD, Drubach DA, Senjem ML, Spychalla AJ, et al. (18)F-FDG PET in posterior cortical atrophy and dementia with Lewy bodies. Journal of Nuclear Medicine. 2017;**58**(4):632-638

[22] Gupta V, Verma R, Ranjan R, Belho ES, Seniaray N, Dinand V, et al. Metabolic imaging patterns in posterior cortical atrophy and Lewy body dementia. Nuclear Medicine Communications. 2019;**40**(12):1275-1282

[23] Hardy CJD, Taylor-Rubin C, Taylor B, Harding E, Gonzalez AS, Jiang J, et al. Symptom-based staging for logopenic variant primary progressive aphasia. European Journal of Neurology. 2024;**31**(7):e16304

[24] Madhavan A, Whitwell JL, Weigand SD, Duffy JR, Strand EA, Machulda MM, et al. FDG PET and MRI in logopenic primary progressive aphasia versus dementia of the Alzheimer's type. PLoS One. 2013;**8**(4):e62471

[25] Nestor PJ, Altomare D, Festari C, Drzezga A, Rivolta J, Walker Z, et al. Clinical utility of FDG-PET for the differential diagnosis among the main forms of dementia. European Journal of Nuclear Medicine and Molecular Imaging. 2018;**45**(9):1509-1525

[26] Bouwman F, Orini S, Gandolfo F, Altomare D, Festari C, Agosta F, et al. Diagnostic utility of FDG-PET in the differential diagnosis between different forms of primary progressive aphasia. European Journal of Nuclear Medicine and Molecular Imaging. 2018;**45**(9):1526-1533

[27] Ossenkoppele R, Prins ND, Pijnenburg YA, Lemstra AW, van der Flier WM, Adriaanse SF, et al. Impact of molecular imaging on the diagnostic process in a memory clinic. Alzheimers Dement. 2013;**9**(4):414-421

[28] Sabri O, Sabbagh MN, Seibyl J, Barthel H, Akatsu H, Ouchi Y, et al. Florbetaben PET imaging to detect amyloid beta plaques in Alzheimer's disease: Phase 3 study. Alzheimers Dement. 2015;**11**(8):964-974

[29] Clark CM, Pontecorvo MJ, Beach TG, Bedell BJ, Coleman RE, Doraiswamy PM, et al. Cerebral PET with florbetapir compared with neuropathology at autopsy for detection of neuritic amyloid-β plaques: A prospective cohort study. Lancet Neurology. 2012;**11**(8):669-678

[30] Burkett BJ, Babcock JC, Lowe VJ, Graff-Radford J, Subramaniam RM, Johnson DR. PET imaging of dementia:

Update 2022. Clinical Nuclear Medicine. 2022;**47**(9):763-773

[31] Kantarci K, Lowe VJ, Chen Q, Przybelski SA, Lesnick TG, Schwarz CG, et al. β-Amyloid PET and neuropathology in dementia with Lewy bodies. Neurology. 2020;**94**(3):e282-e291

[32] Pontecorvo MJ, Devous MD Sr, Navitsky M, Lu M, Salloway S, Schaerf FW, et al. Relationships between flortaucipir PET tau binding and amyloid burden, clinical diagnosis, age and cognition. Brain. 2017;**140**(3):748-763

[33] McKeith IG, Boeve BF, Dickson DW, Halliday G, Taylor JP, Weintraub D, et al. Diagnosis and management of dementia with Lewy bodies: Fourth consensus report of the DLB consortium. Neurology. 2017;**89**(1):88-100

[34] Mukaetova-Ladinska EB, McKeith IG. Pathophysiology of synuclein aggregation in Lewy body disease. Mechanisms of Ageing and Development. 2006;**127**(2):188-202

[35] Oppedal K, Ferreira D, Cavallin L, Lemstra AW, Ten Kate M, Padovani A, et al. A signature pattern of cortical atrophy in dementia with Lewy bodies: A study on 333 patients from the European DLB consortium. Alzheimers Dement. 2019;**15**(3):400-409

[36] Gjerum L, Frederiksen KS, Henriksen OM, Law I, Anderberg L, Andersen BB, et al. A visual rating scale for cingulate island sign on 18F-FDG-PET to differentiate dementia with Lewy bodies and Alzheimer's disease. Journal of the Neurological Sciences. 2020;**410**:116645

[37] Brigo F, Turri G, Tinazzi M. 123I-FP-CIT SPECT in the differential diagnosis between dementia with Lewy bodies and other dementias. Journal of the Neurological Sciences. 2015;**359**(1-2):161-171

[38] Yousaf T, Dervenoulas G, Valkimadi PE, Politis M. Neuroimaging in Lewy body dementia. Journal of Neurology. 2019;**266**(1):1-26

[39] Treglia G, Cason E. Diagnostic performance of myocardial innervation imaging using MIBG scintigraphy in differential diagnosis between dementia with Lewy bodies and other dementias: A systematic review and a meta-analysis. Journal of Neuroimaging. 2012;**22**(2):111-117

[40] Neary D, Snowden JS, Gustafson L, Passant U, Stuss D, Black S, et al. Frontotemporal lobar degeneration: A consensus on clinical diagnostic criteria. Neurology. 1998;**51**(6):1546-1554

[41] Buhour MS, Doidy F, Laisney M, Pitel AL, de La Sayette V, Viader F, et al. Pathophysiology of the behavioral variant of frontotemporal lobar degeneration: A study combining MRI and FDG-PET. Brain Imaging and Behavior. 2017;**11**(1):240-252

[42] Peet BT, Spina S, Mundada N, La Joie R. Neuroimaging in frontotemporal dementia: Heterogeneity and relationships with underlying neuropathology. Neurotherapeutics. 2021;**18**(2):728-752

[43] Matías-Guiu JA, Cabrera-Martín MN, Pérez-Castejón MJ, Moreno-Ramos T, Rodríguez-Rey C, García-Ramos R, et al. Visual and statistical analysis of ^{18}F-FDG PET in primary progressive aphasia. European Journal of Nuclear Medicine and Molecular Imaging. 2015;**42**(6):916-927

[44] Brendel M, Pogarell O, Xiong G, Delker A, Bartenstein P, Rominger A. Depressive symptoms accelerate cognitive

decline in amyloid-positive MCI patients. European Journal of Nuclear Medicine and Molecular Imaging. 2015;**42**(5):716-724

[45] Fu C, Zhang H, Xuan A, Gao Y, Xu J, Shi D. A combined study of (18) F-FDG PET-CT and fMRI for assessing resting cerebral function in patients with major depressive disorder. Experimental and Therapeutic Medicine. 2018;**16**(3):1873-1881

[46] Clergue-Duval V, Questel F, Azuar J, Paquet C, Cognat E, Amami J, et al. Brain 18FDG-PET pattern in patients with alcohol-related cognitive impairment. European Journal of Nuclear Medicine and Molecular Imaging. 2020;**47**(2):281-291

[47] Kuhl DE, Phelps ME, Markham CH, Metter EJ, Riege WH, Winter J. Cerebral metabolism and atrophy in Huntington's disease determined by 18FDG and computed tomographic scan. Annals of Neurology. 1982;**12**(5):425-434

[48] Piccini P, Whone A. Functional brain imaging in the differential diagnosis of Parkinson's disease. Lancet Neurology. 2004;**3**(5):284-290

[49] Hughes AJ, Daniel SE, Ben-Shlomo Y, Lees AJ. The accuracy of diagnosis of parkinsonian syndromes in a specialist movement disorder service. Brain. 2002;**125**(Pt 4):861-870

[50] Darcourt J, Booij J, Tatsch K, Varrone A, Vander Borght T, Kapucu OL, et al. EANM procedure guidelines for brain neurotransmission SPECT using (123)I-labelled dopamine transporter ligands, version 2. European Journal of Nuclear Medicine and Molecular Imaging. 2010;**37**(2):443-450

[51] Quintas S, Sanles-Falagan R, Berbís M. I(123)-FP-CIT (DaTSCAN) SPECT beyond the Most common causes of parkinsonism: A systematic review. Mov Disord Clin Pract. 2024;**11**(6):613-625

[52] Brooks DJ. Imaging approaches to Parkinson disease. Journal of Nuclear Medicine. 2010;**51**(4):596-609

[53] Burn DJ, Sawle GV, Brooks DJ. Differential diagnosis of Parkinson's disease, multiple system atrophy, and Steele-Richardson-Olszewski syndrome: Discriminant analysis of striatal 18F-dopa PET data. Journal of Neurology, Neurosurgery, and Psychiatry. 1994;**57**(3):278-284

[54] Puñal-Riobóo J, Serena-Puig A, Varela-Lema L, Alvarez-Páez AM, Ruano-Ravina A. Clinical utility of (18)F-DOPA-PET in movement disorders. A systematic review. Revista Española de Medicina Nuclear. 2009;**28**(3):106-113

[55] Van Laere K, Varrone A, Booij J, Vander Borght T, Nobili F, Kapucu OL, et al. EANM procedure guidelines for brain neurotransmission SPECT/PET using dopamine D2 receptor ligands, version 2. European Journal of Nuclear Medicine and Molecular Imaging. 2010;**37**(2):434-442

[56] Kim YJ, Ichise M, Ballinger JR, Vines D, Erami SS, Tatschida T, et al. Combination of dopamine transporter and D2 receptor SPECT in the diagnostic evaluation of PD, MSA, and PSP. Movement Disorders. 2002;**17**(2):303-312

[57] Antonini A, Leenders KL, Vontobel P, Maguire RP, Missimer J, Psylla M, et al. Complementary PET studies of striatal neuronal function in the differential diagnosis between multiple system atrophy and Parkinson's disease. Brain. 1997;**120**(12):2187-2195

[58] Verger A, Grimaldi S, Ribeiro MJ, Frismand S, Guedj E. Single photon emission computed tomography/ positron emission tomography molecular imaging for parkinsonism: A fast-developing field. Annals of Neurology. 2021;**90**(5):711-719

[59] Meles SK, Teune LK, de Jong BM, Dierckx RA, Leenders KL. Metabolic imaging in Parkinson disease. Journal of Nuclear Medicine. 2017;**58**(1):23-28

[60] Eckert T, Barnes A, Dhawan V, Frucht S, Gordon MF, Feigin AS, et al. FDG PET in the differential diagnosis of parkinsonian disorders. NeuroImage. 2005;**26**(3):912-921

[61] Zhao P, Zhang B, Gao S. 18F-FDG PET study on the idiopathic Parkinson's disease from several parkinsonian-plus syndromes. Parkinsonism & Related Disorders. 2012;**18**(Suppl. 1):S60-S62

[62] Juh R, Kim J, Moon D, Choe B, Suh T. Different metabolic patterns analysis of parkinsonism on the 18F-FDG PET. European Journal of Radiology. 2004;**51**(3):223-233

[63] Stefanova N, Bücke P, Duerr S, Wenning GK. Multiple system atrophy: An update. Lancet Neurology. 2009;**8**(12):1172-1178

[64] Akdemir Ü, Tokçaer AB, Karakuş A, Kapucu L. Brain 18F-FDG PET imaging in the differential diagnosis of parkinsonism. Clinical Nuclear Medicine. 2014;**39**(3):e220-e226

[65] Ishii K. PET approaches for diagnosis of dementia. AJNR. American Journal of Neuroradiology. 2014;**35**(11):2030-2038

[66] Orimo S, Suzuki M, Inaba A, Mizusawa H. 123I-MIBG myocardial scintigraphy for differentiating Parkinson's disease from other neurodegenerative parkinsonism: A systematic review and meta-analysis. Parkinsonism & Related Disorders. 2012;**18**(5):494-500

[67] Pitton Rissardo J, Fornari Caprara AL. Cardiac 123I-Metaiodobenzylguanidine (MIBG) scintigraphy in Parkinson's disease: A comprehensive review. Brain Sciences. 18 Oct 2023;**13**(10):1471

[68] Vivash L, Gregoire MC, Lau EW, Ware RE, Binns D, Roselt P, et al. 18F-flumazenil: A γ-aminobutyric acid A-specific PET radiotracer for the localization of drug-resistant temporal lobe epilepsy. Journal of Nuclear Medicine. 2013;**54**(8):1270-1277

[69] Ergün EL, Saygi S, Yalnizoglu D, Oguz KK, Erbas B. SPECT-PET in epilepsy and clinical approach in evaluation. Seminars in Nuclear Medicine. 2016;**46**(4):294-307

[70] O'Brien TJ, So EL, Mullan BP, Hauser MF, Brinkmann BH, Bohnen NI, et al. Subtraction ictal SPECT co-registered to MRI improves clinical usefulness of SPECT in localizing the surgical seizure focus. Neurology. 1998;**50**(2):445-454

[71] Kumar A, Chugani HT. The role of radionuclide imaging in epilepsy, part 2: Epilepsy syndromes. Journal of Nuclear Medicine Technology. 2017;**45**(1):22-29

[72] Kikuchi K, Togao O, Yamashita K, Momosaka D, Nakayama T, Kitamura Y, et al. Diagnostic accuracy for the epileptogenic zone detection in focal epilepsy could be higher in FDG-PET/MRI than in FDG-PET/CT. European Radiology. 2021;**31**(5):2915-2922

[73] Zuckier LS, Kolano J. Radionuclide studies in the determination of brain death: Criteria, concepts, and

controversies. Seminars in Nuclear Medicine. 2008;**38**(4):262-273

[74] Abdel-Dayem HM, Bahar RH, Sigurdsson GH, Sadek S, Olivecrona H, Ali AM. The hollow skull: A sign of brain death in Tc-99m HM-PAO brain scintigraphy. Clinical Nuclear Medicine. 1989;**14**(12):912-916

[75] Mrhac L, Zakko S, Parikh Y. Brain death: The evaluation of semi-quantitative parameters and other signs in HMPAO scintigraphy. Nuclear Medicine Communications. 1995;**16**(12):1016-1020

[76] Langen KJ, Herzog H, Kuwert T, Roosen N, Rota E, Kiwit JC, et al. Tomographic studies of rCBF with [99mTc]-HM-PAO SPECT in patients with brain tumors: Comparison with C15O2 continuous inhalation technique and PET. Journal of Cerebral Blood Flow and Metabolism. 1988;**8**(6):S90-S94

[77] Kim KT, Black KL, Marciano D, Mazziotta JC, Guze BH, Grafton S, et al. Thallium-201 SPECT imaging of brain tumors: Methods and results. Journal of Nuclear Medicine. 1990;**31**(6):965-969

[78] Giovacchini G, Riondato M, Giovannini E, Ciarmiello A. Diagnostic applications of nuclear medicine: Brain Tumors. In: Strauss HW, Mariani G, Volterrani D, Larson SM, editors. Nuclear Oncology: From Pathophysiology to Clinical Applications. Cham: Springer International Publishing; 2016. pp. 1-40

[79] Bethge WA, Sandmaier BM. Targeted cancer therapy using radiolabeled monoclonal antibodies. Technology in Cancer Research & Treatment. 2005;**4**(4):393-405

Chapter 4

Clinical Applications of PET/CT in Neuroimaging: Case-Based Approach

Jie Qin, Yang Wu, Xingyu Mu, Jing Ze Li, ZuGuo Li, WeiXia Chong, YuLong Zeng, Lei Zhang, Biyun Mo, Ping Yu and Wei Fu

Abstract

Positron emission tomography/computed tomography (PET/CT) has emerged as a crucial tool in neuroimaging, offering valuable insights into the diagnosis and management of neurological disorders. This chapter explores the clinical applications of PET/CT through a series of case studies, highlighting its role in identifying metabolic and functional alterations in the brain. By analyzing diagnostic images, key imaging features and signal abnormalities that contribute to accurate disease characterization are discussed. Special emphasis is placed on the interpretation of PET/CT findings in conditions such as neurodegenerative diseases, epilepsy, and brain tumors, demonstrating its advantages over conventional imaging techniques. The integration of PET and CT modalities enhances anatomical localization and functional assessment, providing clinicians with critical information for treatment planning. Additionally, emerging advances in radiotracers and quantitative analysis techniques are addressed, underscoring the expanding potential of PET/CT in neuroimaging. This chapter aims to enhance the understanding of PET/CT's diagnostic value, offering insights that bridge research findings with real-world clinical practice.

Keywords: PET/CT, neuroimaging, neurological disorders, diagnostic imaging, metabolic assessment, brain tumors, functional imaging

1. Introduction

Positron emission tomography/computed tomography (PET/CT) has revolutionized neuroimaging by providing both anatomical and functional insights into the brain. This hybrid imaging modality integrates CTs high-resolution anatomical detail with PET's metabolic and molecular information, enabling more precise diagnosis and management of neurological disorders. Compared to conventional imaging techniques such as magnetic resonance imaging (MRI) and standalone CT, PET/CT can detect early physiological changes before structural abnormalities appear, making it a powerful tool in clinical neurology.

PET/CT plays a crucial role in the diagnosis and monitoring of neurodegenerative diseases, epilepsy, and brain tumors. Its ability to detect early pathological changes is particularly valuable in Alzheimer's disease (AD) and Parkinson's disease (PD), aiding in differential diagnosis and disease progression monitoring. Additionally, PET/CT assists in localizing epileptic foci, guiding surgical planning, and characterizing brain tumors to optimize treatment strategies.

The integration of PET and CT enhances anatomical localization and functional assessment, providing clinicians with more comprehensive diagnostic information. However, PET/CT has certain limitations, including radiation exposure, high costs, and limited availability in some regions. Advances in radiotracer development, quantitative imaging techniques, and artificial intelligence-driven image analysis are continuously improving the accuracy and accessibility of PET/CT in neuroimaging.

2. Clinical applications of PET/CT in neuroimaging: Case-based approach

2.1 Postoperative tumor activity assessment of glioblastoma: Comparison between choline and FDG

A female elderly patient was admitted due to a three-month history of headaches and right-sided limb weakness. MRI examination revealed an irregular enhancing signal in the left frontal-temporal region, with poorly defined borders, measuring approximately 3.0 x 2.5 cm. Malignant glioma was suspected. Preoperative systemic evaluation showed no other systemic diseases. On December 1, 2021, the patient underwent craniotomy for tumor resection. Intraoperatively, it was noted that the tumor had indistinct borders with surrounding brain tissue, and parts of the tumor were in close proximity to critical blood vessels and functional areas. A near-total resection was performed. The postoperative pathology report confirmed the diagnosis of glioblastoma (WHO Grade IV). On February 10, 2022, the patient underwent 18F-FDG PET/CT at our hospital, as shown in **Figure 1**.

On February 11, the patient underwent Choline PET/CT, as shown in **Figure 2**.

2.1.1 Discussion

Gliomas, particularly high-grade gliomas such as glioblastoma (WHO Grade IV), have a high postoperative recurrence rate. Early detection of tumor activity is crucial for guiding subsequent treatment. 18F-FDG imaging, as a standard tracer for assessing metabolic activity in various tumors, is limited in brain tumor imaging primarily due to the high background glucose utilization of normal brain tissue [1].

2.1.2 Advantages of choline imaging

Higher Tumor Contrast: Choline, as a marker for cell membrane synthesis, accumulates more in rapidly proliferating tumor cells. Choline PET tracers generally provide higher tumor contrast than FDG, as normal brain tissue has relatively low choline metabolic activity, thus offering better signal contrast for tumors [2].

Lower Background Noise: Due to the low choline transport and phosphatidylcholine synthesis levels in normal brain tissue, Choline PET imaging shows less signal in normal brain regions, helping to more clearly define tumor boundaries and its heterogeneity [3].

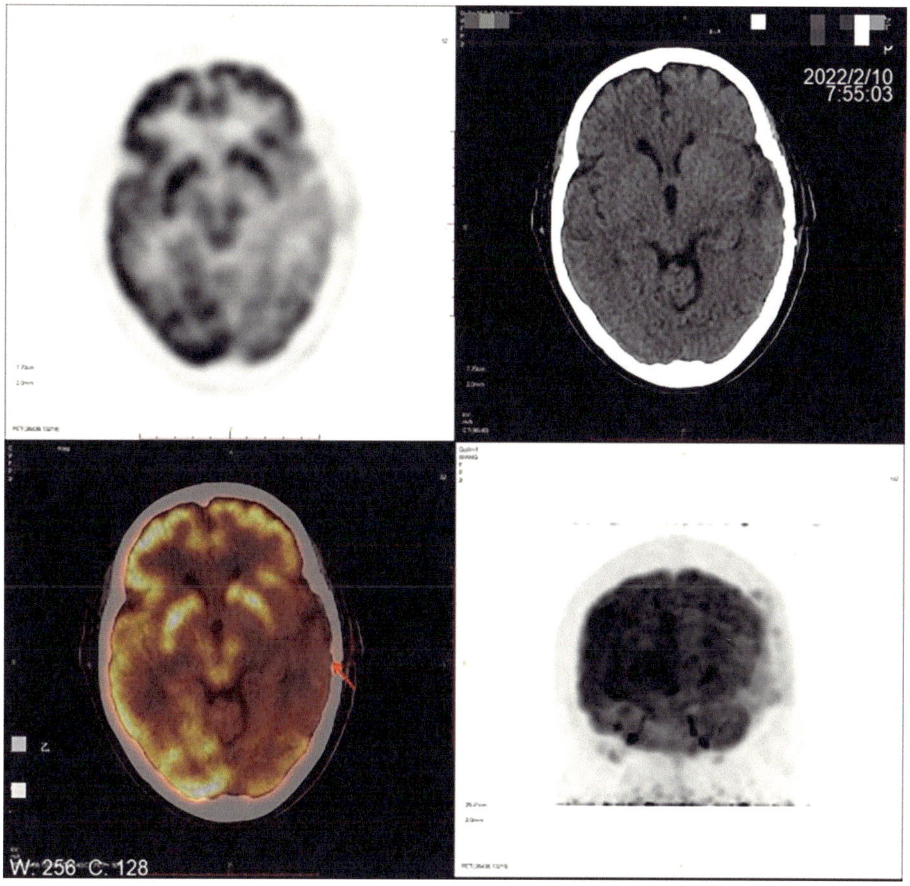

Figure 1.
This figure shows the 18F-FDG PET/CT image of the surgical area, with no observed increase in metabolism. This suggests that there is no significant tumor activity or recurrence in the surgical region, consistent with the expectation of good postoperative local control. The absence of metabolic activity helps exclude tumor recurrence and provides valuable information for subsequent treatment decisions.

Higher Sensitivity and Specificity: Several studies have demonstrated that Choline PET offers higher sensitivity and specificity for detecting residual or recurrent gliomas [4]. Particularly in postoperative evaluations, Choline PET can effectively differentiate between scar tissue and recurrent tumor, which is critical for determining whether further treatment, such as re-surgery or enhanced radiotherapy, is required [5].

2.1.3 Limitations of FDG imaging

High Background Signal: The high uptake of FDG in normal brain tissue leads to increased background signals, which may obscure the signals from tumors with low to moderate metabolic activity, especially when the tumor is near brain gray matter [1].

Diagnostic Ambiguity: The non-specific accumulation of FDG (e.g., inflammation or postoperative changes) may result in false-positive results, affecting the accurate assessment of tumor activity [1].

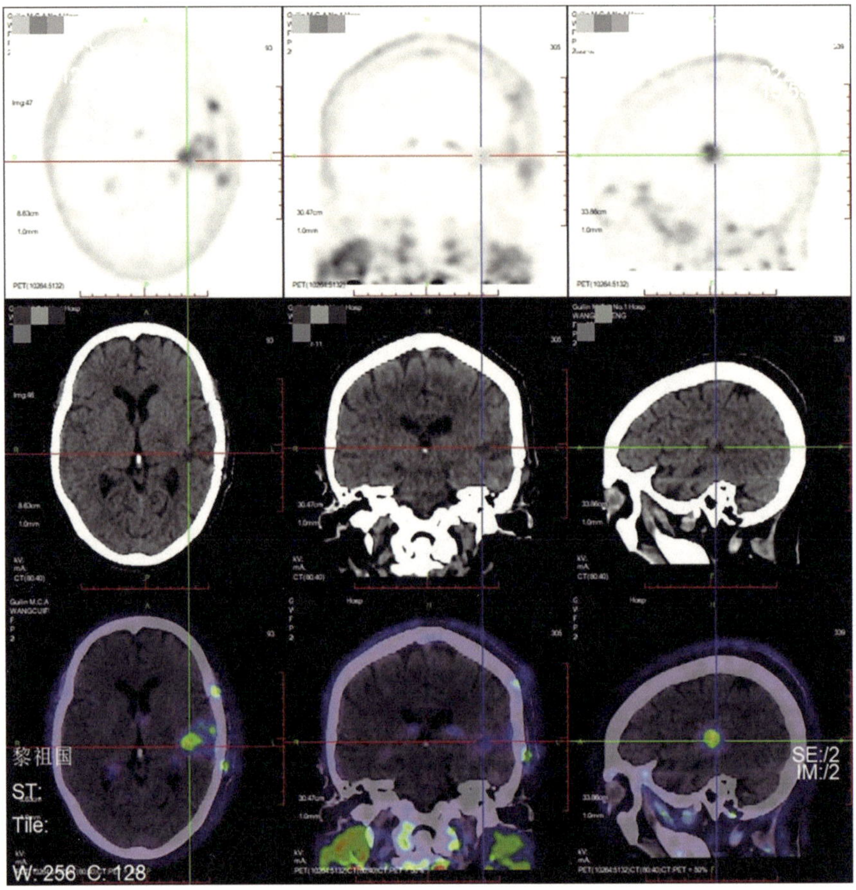

Figure 2.
This figure shows the 18F-DOPA PET/CT image of the surgical area, where increased choline uptake (SUVmax 3.3) is observed. This suggests the presence of tumor tissue or tumor residue in the area, indicating a potential risk of recurrence post-surgery. The increased choline uptake is typically associated with rapidly proliferating tumor cells, providing important clues for subsequent diagnosis and treatment strategies.

2.1.4 Conclusion

Although 18F-FDG remains valuable in diagnosing many types of cancer, Choline PET imaging provides a better option for assessing postoperative tumor activity in glioblastoma. It not only offers more accurate tumor identification but also provides critical information for subsequent treatment decisions by offering higher image contrast and lower background interference [2, 3, 5].

2.2 FDG and DOPA dual-nuclide PET/CT: "The eye of the tiger" reveals Parkinson's disease

A 48-year-old male patient presented with right-hand tremors and bradykinesia for 6 months. He reported that a previous hospital visit suspected Parkinson's disease, with relief after receiving entacapone. In October 2023, an MRI at our hospital showed no abnormalities. He was referred to our department for further evaluation with PET/CT.

DOI: http://dx.doi.org/10.5772/intechopen.1009839

Family History: No family history of hereditary diseases.

Personal History: The patient does not smoke and occasionally drinks alcohol. He has no history of exposure to harmful chemicals in his work environment.

Past Medical History: No history of chronic diseases or neurological disorders.

18F-DOPA PET/CT Imaging on January 3, 2024, in Our Department, as shown in **Figures 3** and **4**.

18F-FDG PET/CT Imaging on January 4, 2024, in our department, as shown in **Figure 5**.

2.2.1 Summary

The application of 18F-DOPA PET imaging in the diagnosis of Parkinson's disease (PD) is a significant area of research. PD is a progressive neurodegenerative disorder

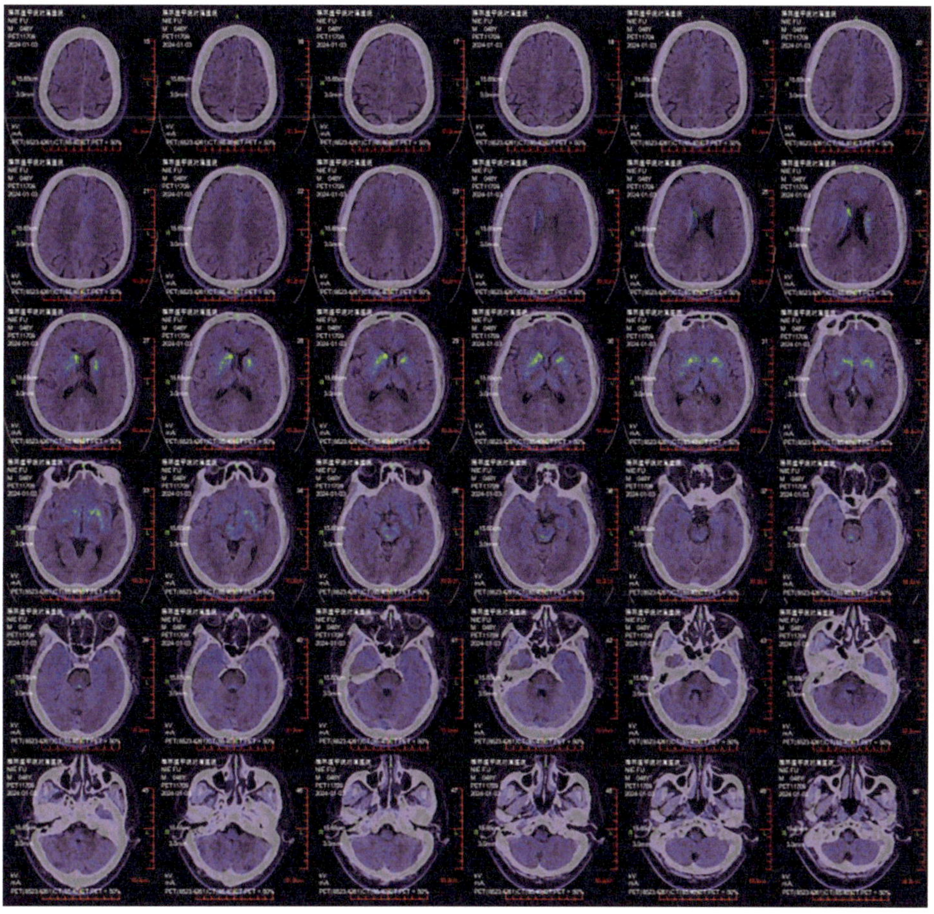

Figure 3.
This figure displays multiple 18F-DOPA PET/CT image slices, showing the metabolic activity in different brain regions. In these slices, you can observe metabolic changes in various regions, including the frontal, parietal, and temporal lobes. The color changes in the images reflect the levels of metabolic activity, with warmer colors (such as red) indicating higher metabolic activity, while cooler colors (such as blue) represent lower metabolic activity. These images are useful for evaluating the brain's metabolic patterns in Parkinson's disease (PD) patients, particularly the changes in the metabolism of the striatum and cerebellum, which are characteristic imaging features of PD.

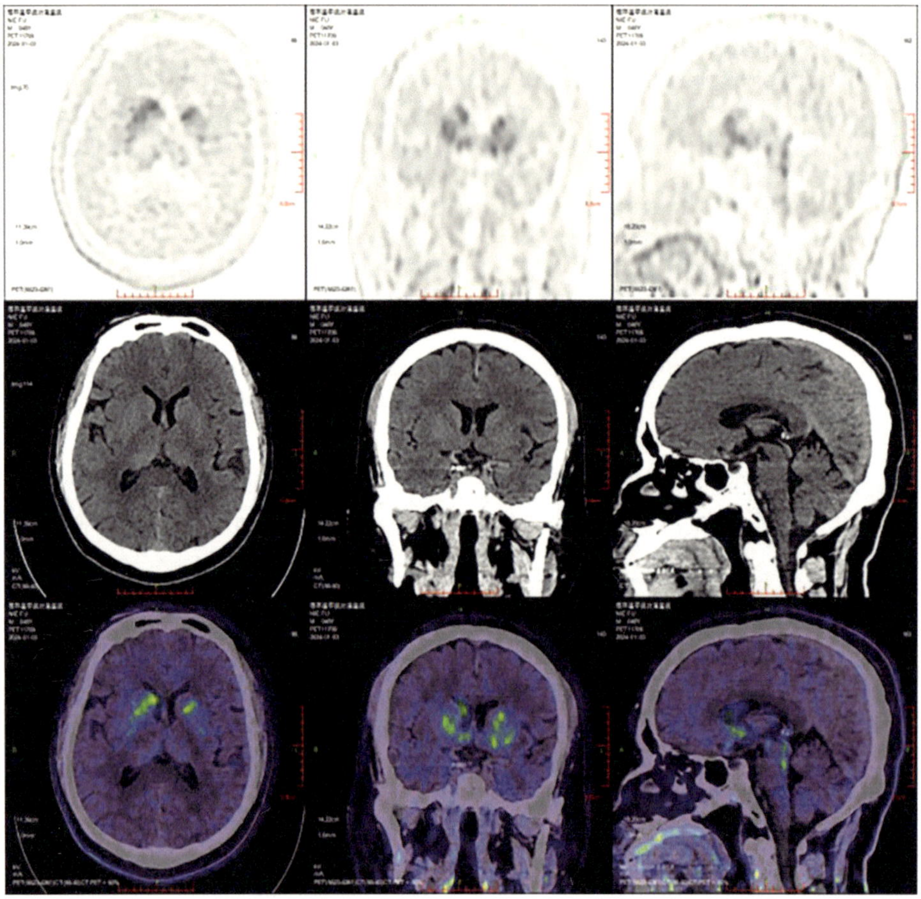

Figure 4.
Reduced 18F-DOPA uptake was observed in the bilateral caudate head, anterior and posterior putamen, with a more significant reduction on the left side, indicating decreased dopamine synthesis.

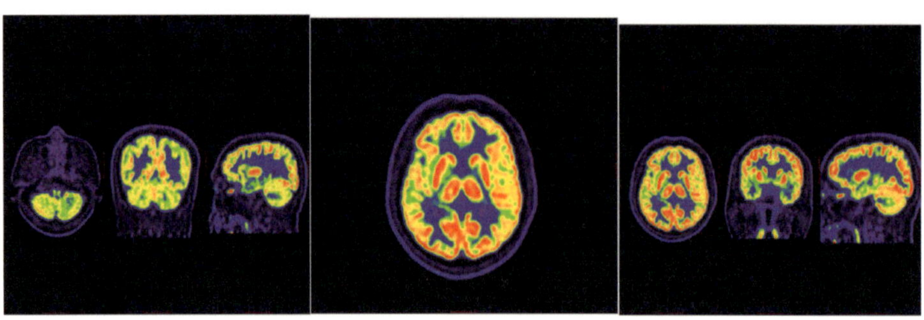

Figure 5.
This figure presents an 18F-FDG PET/CT scan showing increased glucose metabolism in the bilateral caudate nucleus, putamen, and thalamus. These regions are key components of the basal ganglia, which play a central role in motor control and cognitive functions. The elevated metabolic activity observed here is often associated with compensatory mechanisms in Parkinson's disease (PD) or other neurodegenerative disorders. This finding helps differentiate PD from other movement disorders and supports the diagnosis by highlighting characteristic metabolic patterns associated with disease progression.

primarily characterized by motor dysfunction, including tremors, rigidity, bradykinesia, and postural instability [6]. Early diagnosis of PD can be challenging due to the similarity of its early symptoms to other neurological disorders [7].

In this regard, [^18F]DOPA PET imaging provides an effective tool. This technique utilizes [^18F]DOPA, a radiolabeled dopamine precursor, which can be visualized in the brain using PET scanning [8]. In PD patients, dopaminergic neurons in the nigrostriatal pathway degenerate, leading to a decrease in dopamine levels in the brain [9]. Through 18F-DOPA PET imaging, doctors can observe reduced 18F-DOPA uptake in the striatum, which is a typical marker for PD [10]. This reduction correlates with the severity and progression of the disease, making 18F-DOPA PET a valuable tool for early diagnosis and disease monitoring [6, 11]. Additionally, it helps distinguish PD from other movement disorders, such as multiple system atrophy or progressive supranuclear palsy [12].

Throughout the course of PD, certain areas of the brain may show changes in 18F-FDG metabolism, including increased metabolic activity. These changes are often associated with compensatory mechanisms or neuronal responses in affected brain regions [13]. Early in PD, as the brain attempts to compensate for dopaminergic neuron loss, certain areas may exhibit increased metabolism, particularly in the basal ganglia and motor circuits, such as the striatum and pallidum [14]. This phenomenon may reflect an adaptive response to neurotransmitter imbalance. However, as the disease progresses, this increased metabolic activity gradually diminishes, leading to reduced metabolism in later stages [15].

In advanced PD, further neuronal loss and pathological accumulation may result in reduced metabolism in regions such as the frontal cortex, which is linked to cognitive impairment and other non-motor symptoms [16]. It is important to note that 18F-FDG PET/CT is not used for direct PD diagnosis but rather serves as a tool to evaluate brain metabolic activity and assist other diagnostic methods [10].

When both imaging techniques are used together, they provide a more comprehensive neurobiological perspective. By simultaneously evaluating dopamine metabolism and glucose metabolism, clinicians can make a more accurate diagnosis and stage the disease in greater detail [17]. This combined imaging strategy is particularly useful in complex or atypical PD cases, where a single imaging technique may not provide sufficient diagnostic information [12].

2.3 Positive PSMA and OCT imaging in a case of meningioma

A 68-year-old female patient, admitted on October 15, 2022, presented with a history of "bone metastases after thyroid cancer surgery and iodine-131 treatment for two years, accompanied by chest pain and dizziness for 2 months." To assess the patient's overall condition, she underwent 18F-OCT imaging on October 17, as shown in **Figures 6** and 7.

To alleviate thoracic pain, the patient underwent iodine-125 particle implantation for thyroid cancer metastasis to the thoracic vertebra on October 17, 2022. On October 18, the patient requested an 18F-PSMA whole-body scan to reassess the status of her systemic tumors (**Figures 8** and **9**).

2.3.1 Discussion

Meningiomas, originating from arachnoid cap cells, are among the most common primary central nervous system (CNS) tumors, accounting for approximately 37% of

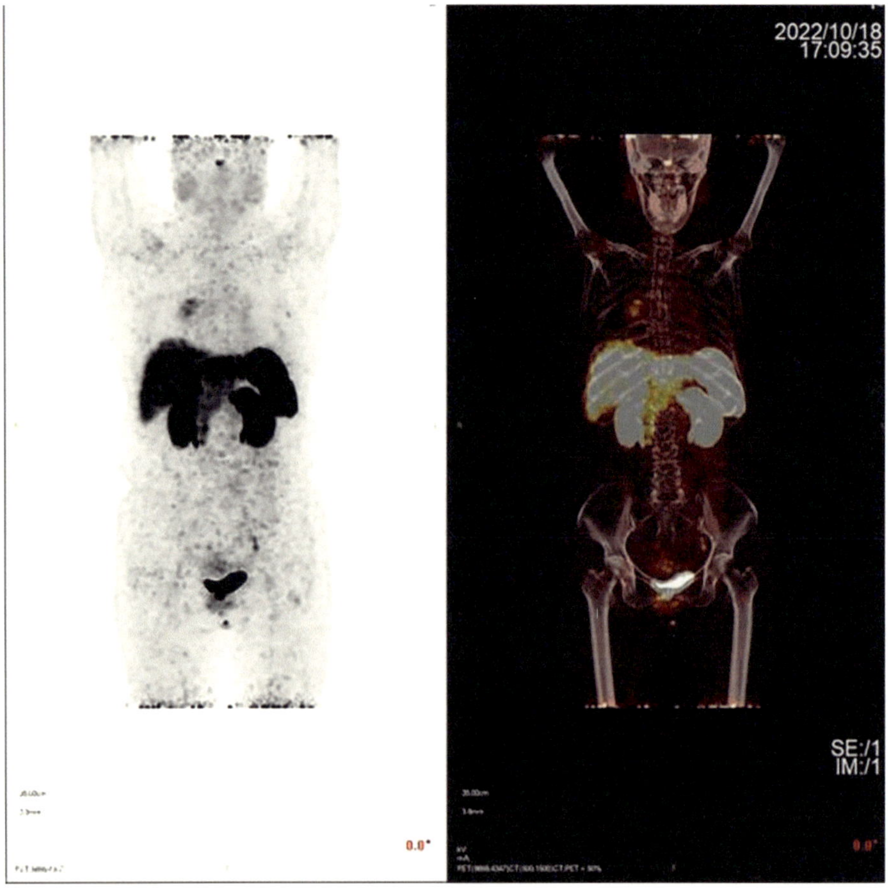

Figure 6.
The scan revealed bone destruction at the T6 vertebra and its attachments, the right 6th posterior rib, and the left femur, with increased somatostatin receptor (octreotide) expression, SUVmax 2.8, suggesting bone metastasis from thyroid cancer.

all brain tumors [18]. They are more prevalent in women, with a male-to-female ratio of about 1:2, and the peak incidence occurs around 45 years of age, while they are rare in children [19].

According to the World Health Organization (WHO), meningiomas are classified into three grades based on histopathological features [20]:

Grade I (Benign): Typically slow-growing, with a low likelihood of recurrence after surgical removal.

Grade II (Atypical): Higher recurrence rates, exhibiting more aggressive behavior.

Grade III (Anaplastic/Malignant): Rare (1–3% of cases), rapid-growing, and highly recurrent.

Approximately 90% of meningiomas occur supratentorially, with common locations including the convexity of the brain, parasagittal region, sphenoid ridge, and olfactory groove [21]. Due to their slow growth, many meningiomas remain asymptomatic and are incidentally discovered during imaging for unrelated conditions [22]. When symptoms appear, they are usually related to the tumor's location, presenting as headaches, seizures, visual disturbances, or motor deficits [23].

DOI: http://dx.doi.org/10.5772/intechopen.1009839

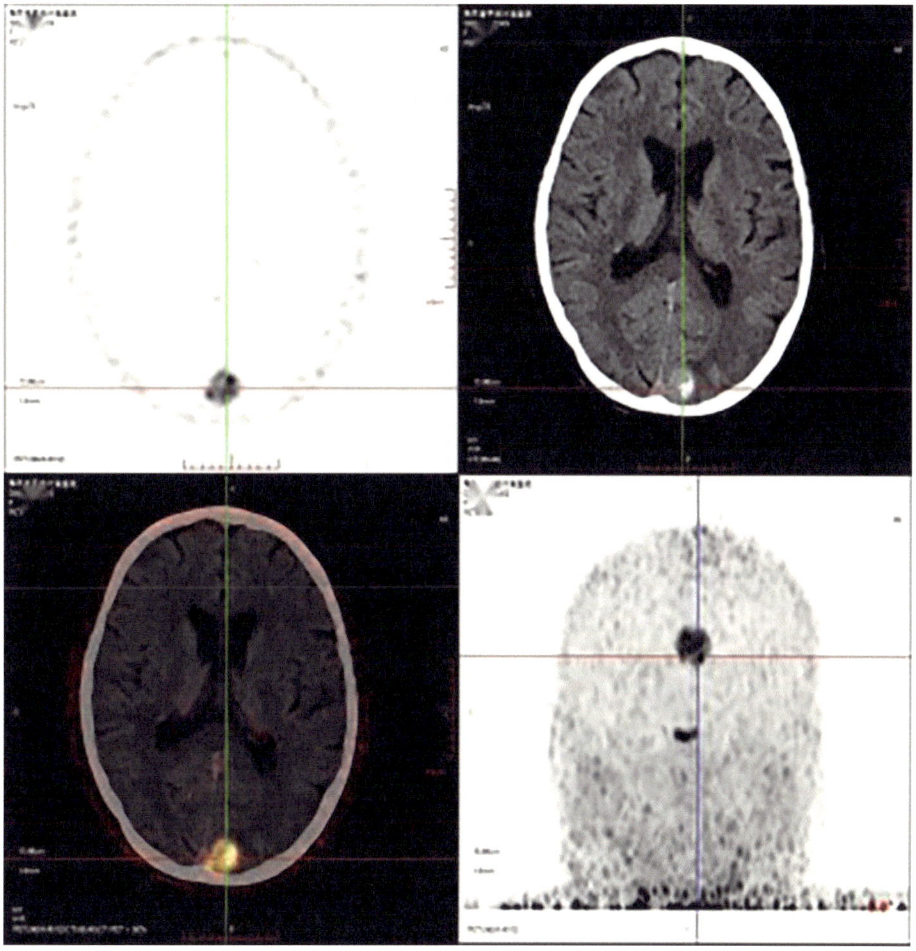

Figure 7.
A slightly high-density, round lesion measuring approximately 17 × 14 mm was observed adjacent to the left occipital region near the falx cerebri. The lesion had clear borders and a broad-based connection to the adjacent bone, with nodular calcifications inside, and no abnormalities were noted in the neighboring bone. PET scan indicated increased radiotracer uptake with an SUVmax of 4.1, further suggesting a meningioma.

2.3.2 Imaging features of meningiomas

Traditional CT and MRI are widely used in diagnosing meningiomas [24]. On non-contrast CT, meningiomas typically appear as well-defined, isodense, or hyperdense masses, sometimes with calcifications. Contrast-enhanced CT reveals homogeneous enhancement with the characteristic "dural tail sign" [25].

2.3.3 Molecular imaging in meningiomas

Recent advancements in molecular imaging have opened new avenues for meningioma evaluation [26]. Prostate-specific membrane antigen (PSMA), a transmembrane glycoprotein first identified in prostate cancer cells, has been found to be expressed in the endothelial cells of neovasculature in non-prostatic tumors,

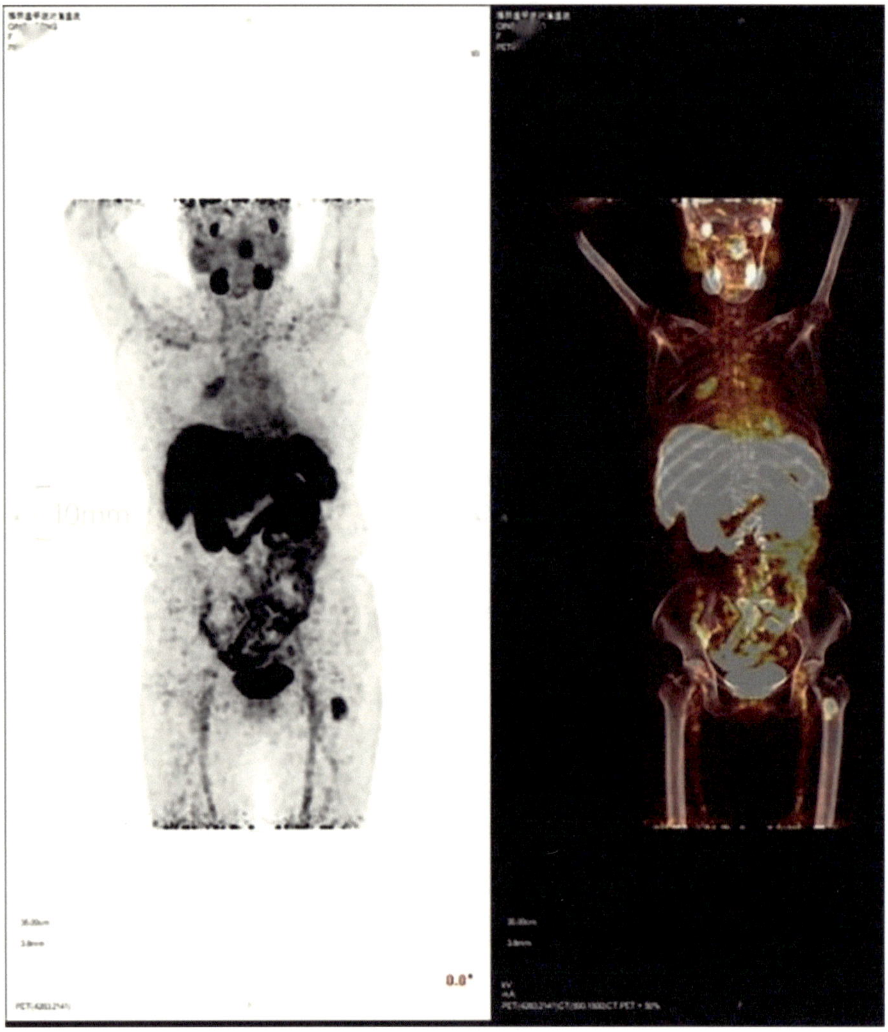

Figure 8.
The scan revealed bone destruction at the T6 vertebra and its attachments, the right 6th posterior rib, and the left femur, with increased PSMA expression, SUVmax 3.7, suggesting bone metastasis from thyroid cancer, with changes following the particle implantation procedure.

including meningiomas [27]. Higher-grade and recurrent meningiomas show increased PSMA expression, making PSMA PET imaging a promising tool for assessing tumor biology and guiding therapeutic strategies [28].

Similarly, somatostatin receptors (SSTRs), particularly subtype 2 (SSTR2), are overexpressed in meningiomas compared to normal brain tissue [29]. This has led to diagnostic imaging applications using radiolabeled somatostatin analogs, such as [^68Ga]DOTATATE PET, which binds specifically to SSTR2 [27]. [^68Ga]DOTATATE PET not only aids in tumor localization but also provides insights into receptor status, which may guide peptide receptor radionuclide therapy (PRRT) [30].

By integrating advanced imaging techniques with traditional pathology, and accumulating large-scale clinical data, we can better understand the relationship between radiotracer uptake patterns and different pathological subtypes of meningiomas [31].

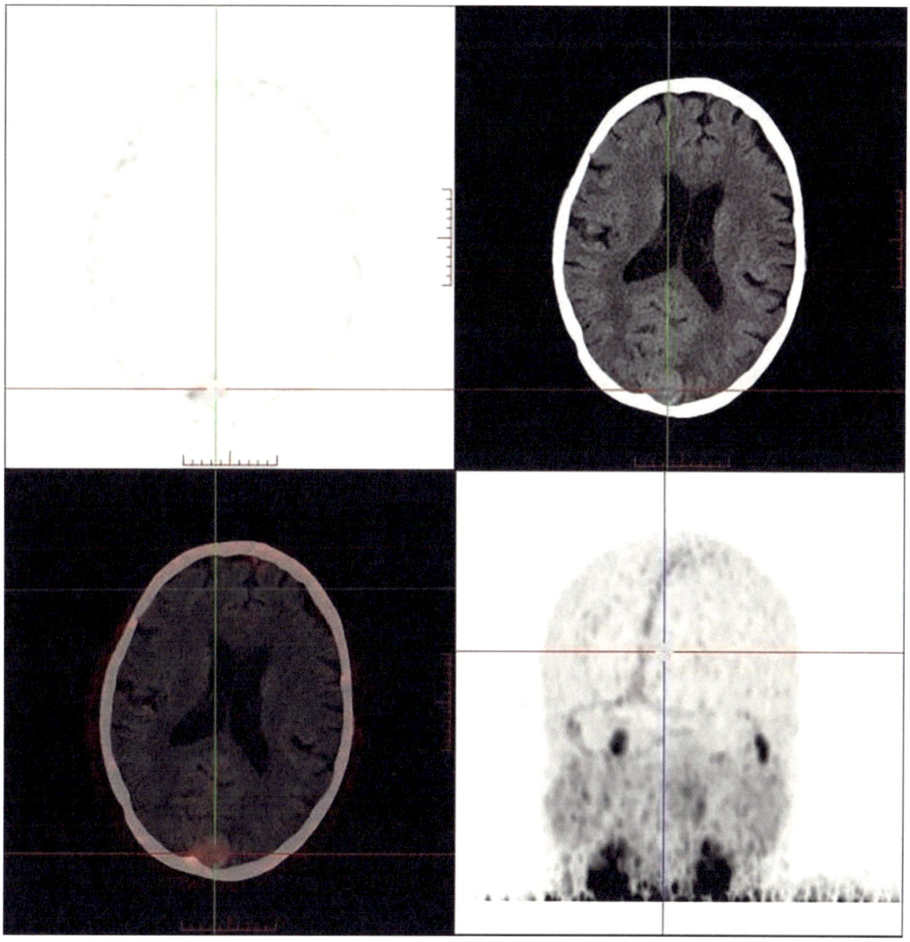

Figure 9.
This image presents the 18F-PSMA PET scan of the brain, with a clear indication of increased radiotracer uptake in the lesion located adjacent to the left occipital region near the falx cerebri. The lesion, measuring approximately 17 × 14 mm, shows elevated PSMA uptake, further supporting the possibility of a meningioma, as previously suggested by the OCT imaging. The PET scan confirms the lesion's metabolic activity, which is consistent with the characteristics of meningiomas that typically exhibit PSMA uptake due to the presence of new vascularity in the tumor. The SUVmax value of 2.0 highlights significant tracer uptake in the region of interest, reinforcing the likelihood of a benign tumor such as meningioma rather than other neoplasms.

This approach enhances diagnostic accuracy and helps develop more effective treatment strategies for both incidental and symptomatic meningiomas [32].

2.4 Postoperative recurrence of pituitary adenoma: Dual-molecular probe PET/CT imaging

A 59-year-old male patient underwent head MRI at a local hospital in 2018 due to dizziness, which suggested a pituitary adenoma. He subsequently underwent a complete resection of the pituitary adenoma. In October 2023, an MRI at another hospital indicated recurrence of the pituitary adenoma, and the patient underwent a second resection. In January 2024, an MRI at another hospital again indicated recurrence of the pituitary adenoma.

Past Medical History: The patient reported significant hypothyroidism post-surgery and was treated with oral levothyroxine sodium tablets for replacement therapy.

The patient was referred for a full-body evaluation with PET/CT, and on March 15, 2024, the 18F-OCT PET/CT results from our hospital were as shown in **Figures 10** and **11**.

To further investigate the lesion, 18F-FAPI-42 imaging was performed, with the following results (**Figures 12** and **13**).

Given these findings, the recurrence of pituitary adenoma is suspected, along with a lesion in the left lobe of the thyroid. Pathological correlation is recommended.

2.4.1 Diagnostic considerations

The pituitary gland, located at the base of the brain, is a crucial part of the endocrine system and is responsible for secreting various hormones that regulate the

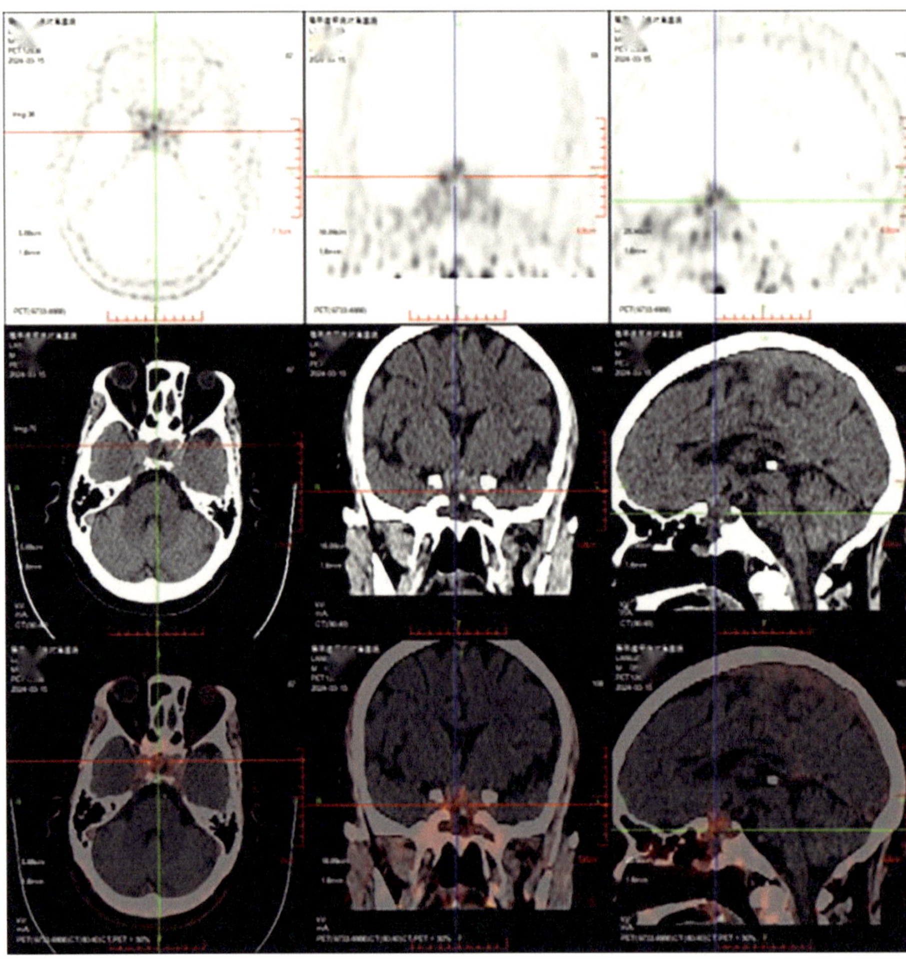

Figure 10.
This figure shows the 18F-OCT PET/CT scan revealing an enlarged sella turcica, approximately 38 × 25 mm in size, with a downward extension through the bony wall of the sphenoid sinus. The SUVmax is 3.5, indicating increased metabolic activity in the pituitary region. This finding is suggestive of pituitary adenoma recurrence and may assist in differentiating it from other sellar-suprasellar lesions. The metabolic activity observed here is crucial for evaluating the potential for tumor recurrence and planning appropriate interventions, such as additional resection or radiotherapy.

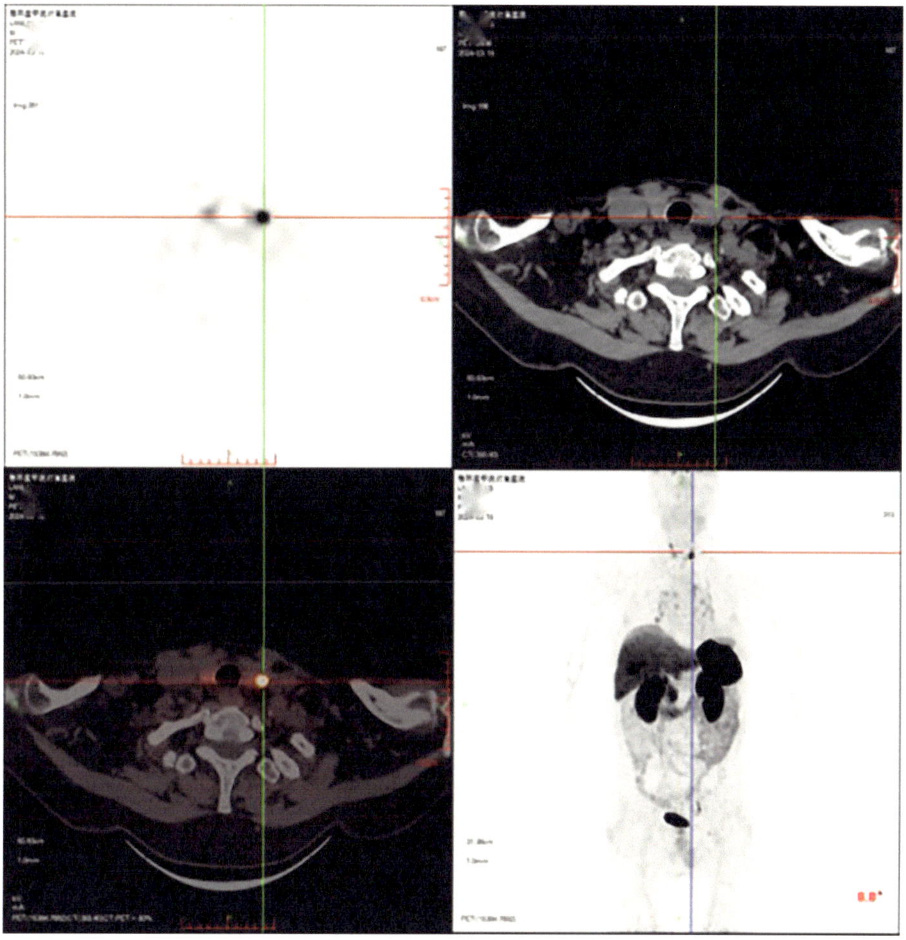

Figure 11.
The thyroid lobes are reduced in size, with a high-density area in the upper pole of the left lobe and uneven density in the lower pole, SUVmax 11.0.

function of other endocrine glands. One of these hormones is thyroid-stimulating hormone (TSH), which stimulates the thyroid to produce thyroid hormones (T3 and T4). These hormones are essential for metabolism, heart function, body temperature regulation, and a range of physiological processes [33].

Pituitary adenomas are tumors that grow abnormally, and while they are often benign, they can compress the pituitary gland as they increase in size, disrupting its normal function. If a pituitary adenoma affects the gland's ability to secrete TSH, this can lead to reduced stimulation of the thyroid, thereby decreasing the production and secretion of thyroid hormones. This type of hypothyroidism caused by pituitary dysfunction is referred to as central hypothyroidism, which differs from primary hypothyroidism caused by a dysfunction within the thyroid itself [34].

In this case, one possible diagnosis is the recurrence of the pituitary adenoma: The high expression on OCT imaging suggests the recurrence of the pituitary tumor [35]. Some pituitary adenoma cells may express somatostatin receptors, which can be captured through OCT imaging [36]. Additionally, the high expression on FAPI imaging may reflect pathological changes in the pituitary area post-surgery, such as fibrosis or

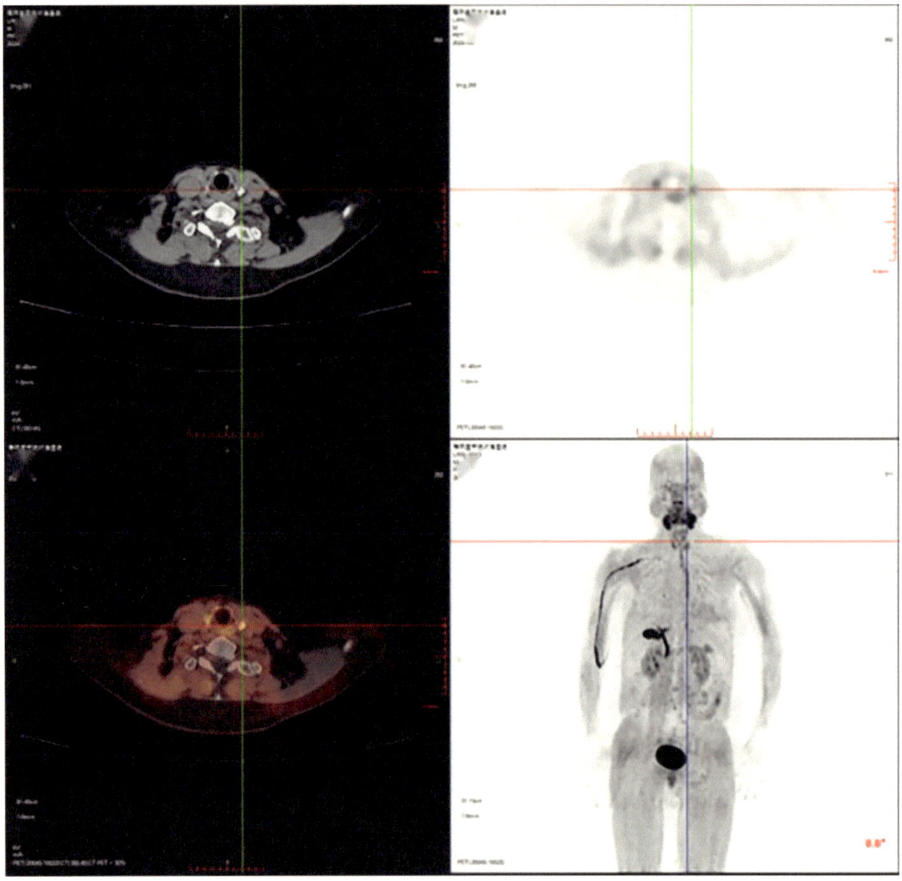

Figure 12.
The thyroid lobes are reduced in size, with a high-density area in the upper pole of the left lobe and uneven density in the lower pole, SUVmax 4.4.

increased cellular activity of the tumor cells. Comprehensive evaluation of pituitary function, including the measurement of pituitary hormone levels, is recommended to determine whether there is dysfunction of the anterior or posterior pituitary gland [37, 38].

2.5 18F-DOPA and 18F-FDG imaging in the diagnosis of multiple system atrophy: A case report

A 50-year-old female patient was admitted due to "right-sided limb bradykinesia for over a year." The patient reported that about a year ago, she noticed bradykinesia in her right limbs, mainly presenting as difficulty holding a pen and chopsticks, as well as difficulty lifting her right lower limb while walking. She also experienced difficulty with speech articulation. She is still able to manage daily activities independently, but the symptoms have progressively worsened over the past 6 months. She presented to our hospital for further evaluation and treatment.

Laboratory Tests: Routine blood and urine tests, liver and kidney function, and tumor markers showed no significant abnormalities.

Imaging Studies: MRI showed involvement in the right basal ganglia, right temporo-occipital-parietal region, and bilateral frontal white matter areas.

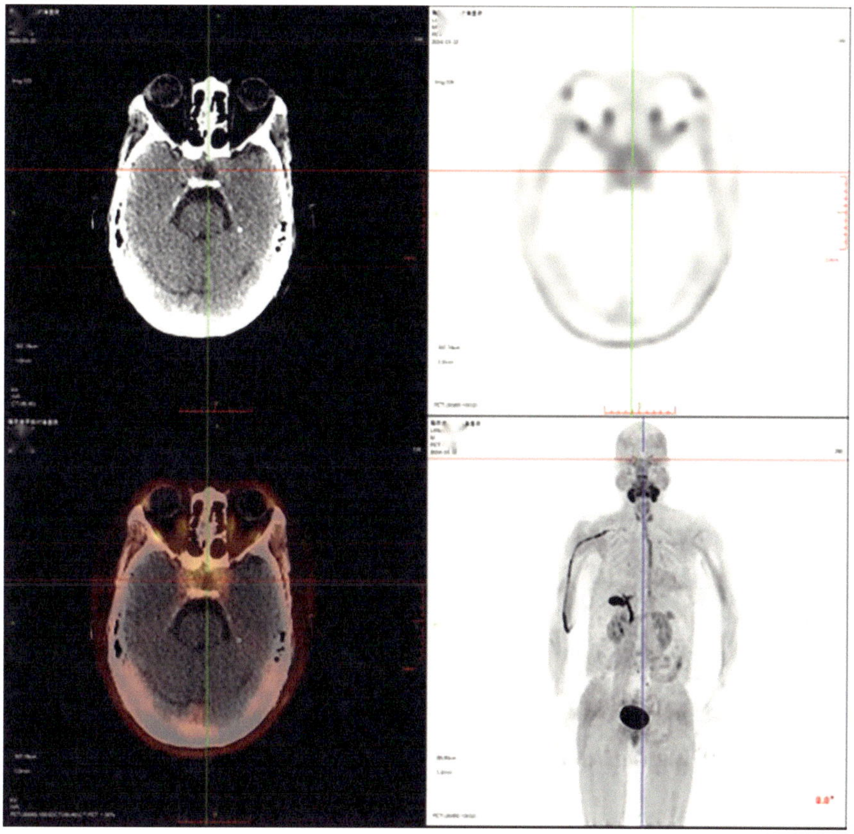

Figure 13.
The sella turcica is enlarged, measuring approximately 38 × 25 mm, with downward extension through the bony wall of the sphenoid sinus, SUVmax 3.2.

To further investigate the lesion, 18F-DOPA imaging was performed, with the following results (**Figure 14**).

18F-FDG imaging was performed, with the following results (**Figure 15**).

Multiple system atrophy (MSA) is a progressive neurodegenerative disorder that typically manifests between ages 40 and 60. Its exact cause remains unclear, though research suggests a combination of genetic predisposition, environmental influences, and neurodegenerative changes [39]. Clinically, MSA is characterized by autonomic dysfunction, Parkinsonism, and cerebellar ataxia, often presenting together and complicating diagnosis. MSA is classified into two subtypes: Parkinsonian type (MSA-P) and cerebellar type (MSA-C) [40].

2.5.1 Pathological characteristics

MSA is marked by degeneration of the dopaminergic system, particularly in the basal ganglia and cerebellum, contributing to its motor symptoms [41].

MSA-P patients primarily exhibit Parkinsonian features, with some cerebellar involvement. Their FDG metabolism pattern typically shows reduced glucose metabolism in the bilateral striatum, especially in the posterior putamen, along with cerebellar hypometabolism [41].

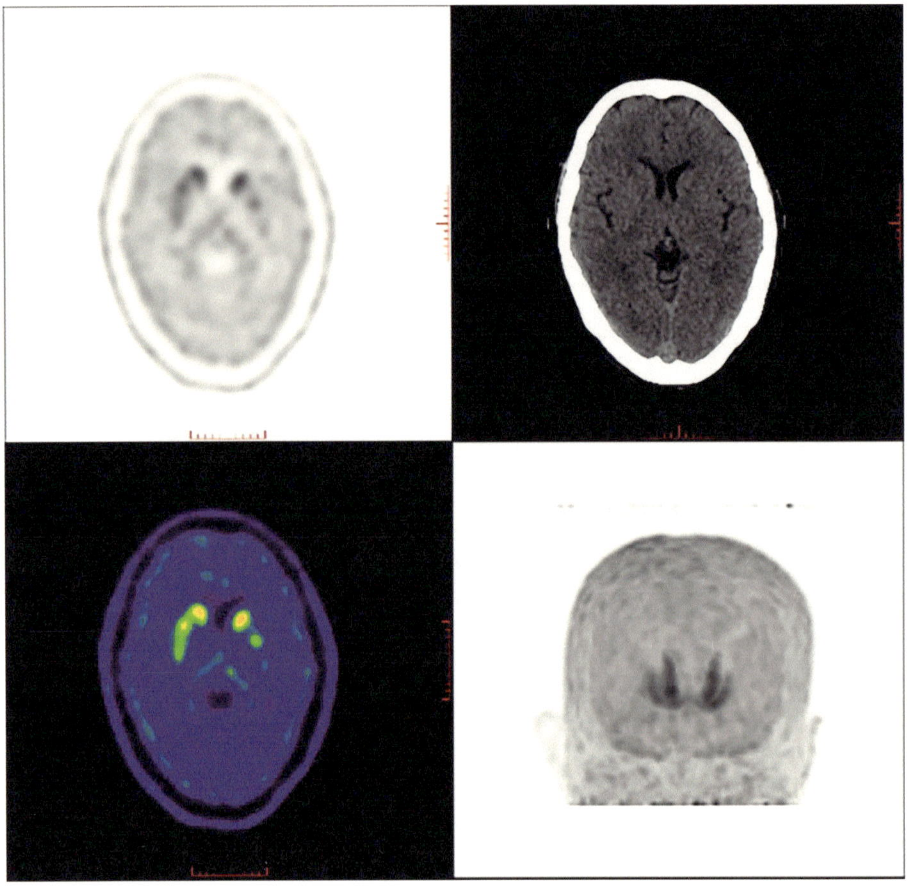

Figure 14.
Reduced 18F-DOPA uptake was observed in the bilateral caudate head, as well as the anterior and posterior putamen, indicating decreased dopamine synthesis. This pattern is characteristic of multiple system atrophy (MSA), a neurodegenerative disorder marked by dopaminergic dysfunction. The reduced uptake reflects the degeneration of dopaminergic neurons, which contributes to the motor and autonomic symptoms seen in MSA. This imaging finding plays a crucial role in differentiating MSA from other movement disorders, such as Parkinson's disease, by highlighting the extent and distribution of dopaminergic deficits.

MSA-C predominantly affects the cerebellum, with significant cerebellar hypometabolism, whereas striatal metabolism is only mildly reduced or remains normal [41].

2.5.2 Imaging characteristics

Both 18F-DOPA and 18F-FDG PET imaging play crucial roles in the early diagnosis and differentiation of MSA [42].

18F-DOPA PET assesses dopamine synthesis and reveals reduced uptake in the bilateral caudate head, anterior and posterior putamen, indicative of dopaminergic degeneration characteristic of MSA [42].

18F-FDG PET reflects metabolic alterations, typically showing decreased metabolism in the bilateral striatum (particularly the posterior putamen) and cerebellum [43].

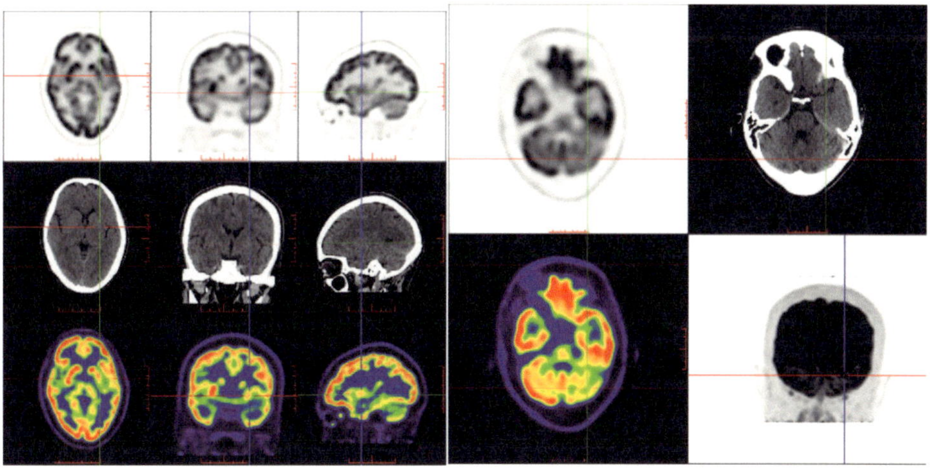

Figure 15.
18F-FDG Imaging: Reduced FDG metabolism was observed in the left temporal lobe, posterior putamen on the left, and the left cerebellar hemisphere.

MSA-P presents with metabolic deficits in both the basal ganglia and cerebellum [43].

MSA-C exhibits predominant cerebellar hypometabolism, with only mild or no involvement of the striatum [43].

2.5.3 Clinical diagnosis and differentiation

Integrating 18F-DOPA and 18F-FDG PET findings enhances the accuracy of MSA diagnosis and its subtype classification [44]. These imaging techniques are instrumental in differentiating MSA from other neurodegenerative disorders, guiding treatment strategies, and monitoring disease progression [45].

2.6 18F-AV45 PET/CT imaging: A case report

A 74-year-old female patient with a 4-year history of progressive memory decline, primarily affecting recent memory. Her ability to perform daily activities is still intact. She previously underwent total thyroidectomy for thyroid cancer and has no history of hypertension, diabetes, or other diseases.

The patient was referred for auxiliary diagnosis to determine if Alzheimer's disease (AD) is the cause. She underwent 18F-AV45 PET/CT brain metabolic imaging at our department. 18F-AV45 imaging was performed, with the following results (**Figure 16**).

2.6.1 Summary

Alzheimer's disease (AD) is a neurodegenerative disorder characterized by progressive cognitive decline, accompanied by behavioral and psychiatric abnormalities, ultimately leading to a loss of daily living abilities [46]. The hallmark pathological changes include the deposition of beta-amyloid (Aβ) plaques and the formation of neurofibrillary tangles [46]. AD is the most common form of dementia in the elderly, severely impacting the physical and mental health of middle-aged and elderly individuals and placing a heavy burden on families and society [47].

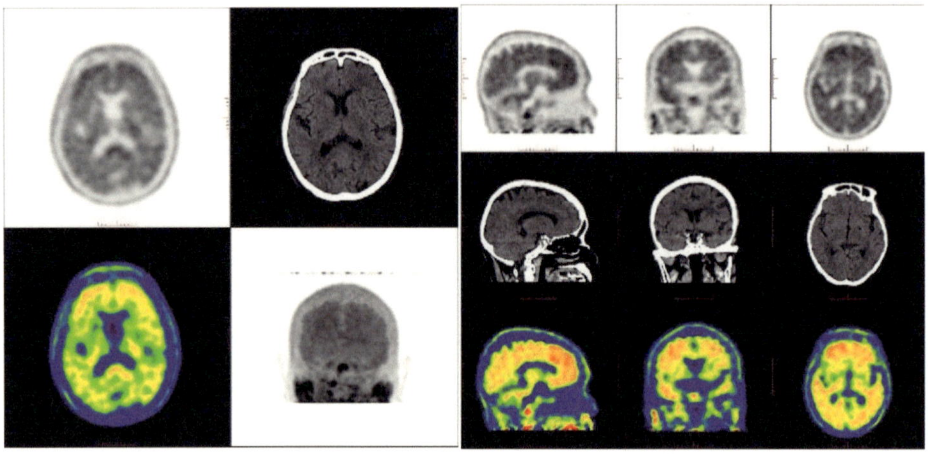

Figure 16.
18F-AV45 PET/CT results showed increased uptake of 18F-AV45 in the bilateral parietal, frontal, temporal lobes, and posterior cingulate gyrus, indicating widespread amyloid deposition, which was positive for amyloid plaque imaging.

2.6.2 18F-AV45 PET imaging in AD diagnosis

18F-AV45, as an Aβ PET imaging agent, can quantify the deposition of amyloid plaques in the brains of AD patients [48]. Currently, amyloid PET has been accepted as part of the AD diagnostic process and is used as a clinical and research standard for AD diagnosis [49]. Studies have reported that the sensitivity and specificity of Aβ deposition in AD patients can reach 96% and 100%, respectively [50].

Subjective cognitive decline (SCD) refers to self-perceived cognitive decline without objective impairment, but it increases the risk of progressing to mild cognitive impairment (MCI) and Alzheimer's disease (AD) [51]. Amyloid deposition in the brain can also be observed in SCD patients [52].

2.6.3 Aβ-positive imaging features and clinical implications

Typical Aβ-positive imaging features include a significant reduction in the contrast between gray and white matter uptake due to increased gray matter uptake [53]. In this case, 18F-AV45 imaging showed significant positive changes [54]. However, a comprehensive evaluation, including cognitive assessments, is needed to confirm whether this is AD [55].

2.6.4 Summary

The Application of PET/CT Imaging in Neurological Disease Diagnosis.

This chapter presents a series of clinical cases demonstrating the crucial role of PET/CT imaging in diagnosing neurological disorders. Firstly, in the postoperative assessment of glioblastoma recurrence, Choline PET/CT exhibited superior tumor contrast and sensitivity compared to 18F-FDG PET/CT, effectively distinguishing between tumor recurrence and postoperative scar tissue. This distinction is essential for guiding further treatment strategies. Secondly, in the diagnosis of Parkinson's disease (PD), 18F-DOPA PET/CT effectively evaluates dopamine metabolism in the nigrostriatal pathway by detecting reduced dopamine uptake in the caudate nucleus and putamen. This imaging modality helps differentiate PD from other movement disorders such as multiple system atrophy (MSA) or progressive supranuclear palsy (PSP). Additionally, 18F-FDG PET/CT can reveal compensatory hypermetabolism in early PD and hypometabolism in advanced PD, aiding in disease staging and progression monitoring.

For meningiomas, PSMA PET/CT and OCT PET/CT demonstrated high uptake, indicating the molecular characteristics of these tumors. PSMA expression is elevated in higher-grade or recurrent meningiomas, making it a potential imaging and therapeutic target, while OCT imaging, through somatostatin receptor (SSTR) expression, provides an alternative approach for precise imaging and treatment guidance. In the evaluation of recurrent pituitary adenoma, OCT PET/CT demonstrated high uptake, suggesting the expression of somatostatin receptors in tumor cells. Additionally, FAPI PET/CT indicated increased uptake in postoperative regions, suggesting fibrosis or enhanced cellular activity, which aids in assessing postoperative recurrence. A comprehensive evaluation of pituitary hormone function, combined with imaging findings, enhances the early detection of pituitary adenoma recurrence. For multiple system atrophy (MSA), the combined application of 18F-DOPA PET/CT and 18F-FDG PET/CT is invaluable in distinguishing MSA subtypes (MSA-P vs. MSA-C). 18F-DOPA PET/CT detects dopaminergic degeneration in the nigrostriatal pathway, while 18F-FDG PET/CT reveals metabolic abnormalities in the basal ganglia and cerebellum, improving diagnostic accuracy and differentiation from PD or PSP. Finally, in the diagnosis of Alzheimer's disease (AD), 18F-AV45 PET/CT demonstrated widespread amyloid deposition, confirming the presence of Aβ plaques, a hallmark of AD. Amyloid PET imaging plays a crucial role in distinguishing AD from other dementias, such as frontotemporal dementia (FTD) or dementia with Lewy bodies (DLB). It also allows for monitoring of disease progression and assessing anti-amyloid therapies.

2.6.5 Future perspectives

This chapter highlights the versatile applications of PET/CT imaging in neurological diseases, covering brain tumors, Parkinson's disease, multiple system atrophy, and Alzheimer's disease. The combination of various molecular probes (FDG, DOPA, AV45, choline, PSMA, FAPI, and OCT) provides high-resolution imaging for early diagnosis, disease classification, progression monitoring, and postoperative recurrence assessment. As molecular imaging and AI-assisted imaging analysis continue to advance, PET/CT will play an increasingly significant role in precision medicine for neurological disorders. Future research should focus on multimodal PET integration (e.g., PET/MRI), the development of higher-affinity radiotracers, quantitative imaging analysis, and the exploration of radiopharmaceutical-targeted therapy (e.g., PRRT for meningiomas). These advancements will further enhance the clinical value of PET/CT in diagnosing and managing neurological diseases.

Acknowledgements

We would like to express our sincere gratitude to the medical and research teams who contributed to the imaging studies and clinical analyses presented in this chapter. Special thanks go to the nuclear medicine department for their expertise in PET/CT imaging and data interpretation. We also appreciate the support from our institution and funding bodies that have facilitated this research. Lastly, we extend our heartfelt appreciation to the patients and their families for their participation and trust, which have made this work possible.

The author acknowledges the use of ChatGPT (OpenAI) for language polishing of the manuscript.

Author details

Jie Qin[1], Yang Wu[1], Xingyu Mu[1], Jing Ze Li[1], ZuGuo Li[1], WeiXia Chong[1], YuLong Zeng[1], Lei Zhang[1], Biyun Mo[1], Ping Yu[2] and Wei Fu[1]*

1 Department of Nuclear Medicine, The First Affiliated Hospital of Guilin Medical University, Guilin, China

2 Department of Endocrinology, The First Affiliated Hospital of Guilin Medical University, Guilin, China

*Address all correspondence to: fuwei19700513@163.com

References

[1] Hara T, Kosaka N, Shinoura N, Kondo T. PET imaging of brain tumor with [methyl-11C]choline. Journal of Nuclear Medicine. 1997;**38**(6):842-847. Available from: https://pubmed.ncbi.nlm.nih.gov/9189127/

[2] Kato T, Shinoda J, Nakayama N, Miwa K, Okumura A, Yano H, et al. Metabolic assessment of gliomas using 11C-methionine, [18F] fluorodeoxyglucose, and 11C-choline positron-emission tomography. AJNR. American Journal of Neuroradiology. 2008;**29**(6):1176-1182. DOI: 10.3174/ajnr.A1008

[3] Takenaka S, Asano Y, Shinoda J, Nomura Y, Yonezawa S, Miwa K, et al. Comparison of 11C-methionine, 11C-choline, and 18F-FDG-PET for distinguishing glioma recurrence from radiation necrosis. Neurologia Medico-Chirurgica. 2014;**54**(4):280-289. DOI: 10.2176/nmc.oa2013-0117

[4] Wyss MT, Spaeth N, Biollaz G, Pahnke J, Alessi P, Trachsel E, et al. Uptake of 18F-fluorocholine, 18F-FET, and 18F-FDG in C6 gliomas and correlation with 131I-SIP(L19), a marker of angiogenesis. Journal of Nuclear Medicine. 2007;**48**(4):608-614. DOI: 10.2967/jnumed.106.036251

[5] Gao L, Xu W, Li T, Zheng J, Chen G. Accuracy of 11C-choline positron emission tomography in differentiating glioma recurrence from radiation necrosis: A systematic review and meta-analysis. Medicine (Baltimore). 2018;**97**(29):e11556. DOI: 10.1097/MD.0000000000011556

[6] Darcourt J, Schiazza A, Sapin N, Dufour M, Ouvrier MJ, Benisvy D, et al. 18F-FDOPA PET for the diagnosis of parkinsonian syndromes. The Quarterly Journal of Nuclear Medicine and Molecular Imaging. 2014;**58**(4):355-365. Epub 2014 Nov 4

[7] Brooks DJ, Pavese N. Imaging biomarkers in Parkinson's disease. Progress in Neurobiology. 2011;**95**(4):614-628. DOI: 10.1016/j.pneurobio.2011.08.009. Epub 2011 Aug 30

[8] Pavese N, Brooks DJ. Imaging neurodegeneration in Parkinson's disease. Biochimica et Biophysica Acta. 2009;**1792**(7):722-729. DOI: 10.1016/j.bbadis.2008.10.003

[9] Eidelberg D. Metabolic brain networks in neurodegenerative disorders: A functional imaging approach. Trends in Neurosciences. 2005;**28**(10):548-560. DOI: 10.1016/j.tins.2009.05.003

[10] Tang CC, Poston KL, Dhawan V, Eidelberg D. Abnormalities in metabolic network activity precede the onset of motor symptoms in Parkinson's disease. The Journal of Neuroscience. 2010;**30**(3):1049-1056. DOI: 10.1523/JNEUROSCI.4188-09.2010

[11] Antonini A, Tolosa E, Mizuno Y, Yamamoto M, Poewe WH. A reassessment of risks and benefits of dopamine agonists in Parkinson's disease. Lancet Neurology. 2009;**8**(10):929-937. DOI: 10.1016/S1474-4422(09)70225-X. Epub 2009 Aug 24

[12] Meyer PT, Frings L, Rücker G, Hellwig S. 18F-FDG PET in parkinsonism: Differential diagnosis and evaluation of cognitive impairment. Journal of Nuclear Medicine. 2017;**58**(12):1888-1898. DOI: 10.2967/jnumed.116.186403. Epub 2017 Sep 14

[13] Eckert T, Eidelberg D. Neuroimaging and therapeutics in movement disorders. NeuroRx. 2005;**2**(2):361-371. DOI: 10.1602/neurorx.2.2.361

[14] Varrone A, Halldin C. New developments of dopaminergic imaging in Parkinson's disease. The Quarterly Journal of Nuclear Medicine and Molecular Imaging. 2012;**56**(1): 68-82

[15] Bohnen NI, Djang DS, Herholz K, Anzai Y, Minoshima S. Effectiveness and safety of 18F-FDG PET in the evaluation of dementia: A review of the recent literature. Journal of Nuclear Medicine. 2012;**53**(1):59-71. DOI: 10.2967/jnumed.111.096578. Epub 2011 Dec 15

[16] Huang C, Mattis P, Tang C, Perrine K, Carbon M, Eidelberg D. Metabolic brain networks associated with cognitive function in Parkinson's disease. NeuroImage. 2007;**34**(2):714-723. ISSN 1053-8119. DOI: 10.1016/j.neuroimage.2006.09.003

[17] Eggers C, Schwartz F, Pedrosa DJ, Kracht L, Timmermann L. Parkinson's disease subtypes show a specific link between dopaminergic and glucose metabolism in the striatum. PLoS One. 2014;**9**(5):e96629. DOI: 10.1371/journal.pone.0096629

[18] Ostrom QT, Price M, Neff C, Cioffi G, Waite KA, Kruchko C, et al. CBTRUS statistical report: Primary brain and other central nervous system tumors diagnosed in the United States in 2015-2019. Neuro-Oncology. 2022;**24**(Suppl 5):v1-v95. DOI: 10.1093/neuonc/noac202

[19] Louis DN, Perry A, Reifenberger G, von Deimling A, Figarella-Branger D, Cavenee WK, et al. The 2016 World Health Organization classification of tumors of the central nervous system: A summary. Acta Neuropathologica. 2016;**131**(6):803-820. DOI: 10.1007/s00401-016-1545-1. Epub 2016 May 9

[20] Goldbrunner R, Stavrinou P, Jenkinson MD, Sahm F, Mawrin C, Weber DC, et al. EANO guideline on the diagnosis and management of meningiomas. Neuro-Oncology. 2021;**23**(11):1821-1834. DOI: 10.1093/neuonc/noab150

[21] Sun C, Dou Z, Wu J, Jiang B, Iranmanesh Y, Yu X, et al. The preferred locations of meningioma according to different biological characteristics based on voxel-wise analysis. Frontiers in Oncology. 2020;**10**:1412. DOI: 10.3389/fonc.2020.01412

[22] Mawrin C, Perry A. Pathological classification and molecular genetics of meningiomas. Journal of Neuro-Oncology. 2010;**99**(3):379-391. DOI: 10.1007/s11060-010-0342-2. Epub 2010 Sep 1

[23] Alruwaili AA, De Jesus O. Meningioma. In: StatPearls [Internet]. Treasure Island (FL): StatPearls Publishing; 2025. Available from: https://www.ncbi.nlm.nih.gov/books/NBK560538/?utm_source=chatgpt.com [Accessed: August 23, 2023]

[24] García Garzón JR, de Arcocha Torres M, Delgado-Bolton R, Ceci F, Alvarez Ruiz S, Orcajo Rincón J, et al. 68Ga-PSMA PET/CT in prostate cancer. Revista Española de Medicina Nuclear e Imagen Molecular (English Edition). 2018;**37**(2):130-138. English, Spanish. DOI: 10.1016/j.remn.2017.07.004. Epub 2017 Sep 21

[25] Rachinger W, Stoecklein VM, Terpolilli NA, Haug AR, Ertl L, Pöschl J, et al. Increased 68Ga-DOTATATE uptake in PET imaging discriminates meningioma and tumor-free tissue. Journal of Nuclear Medicine.

2015;**56**(3):347-353. DOI: 10.2967/jnumed.114.149120. Epub 2015 Jan 29

[26] Mirian C, Duun-Henriksen AK, Maier A, Pedersen MM, Jensen LR, Bashir A, et al. Somatostatin receptor-targeted radiopeptide therapy in treatment-refractory meningioma: Individual patient data meta-analysis. Journal of Nuclear Medicine. 2021;**62**(4):507-513. DOI: 10.2967/jnumed.120.249607. Epub 2020 Aug 28

[27] Reubi JC, Waser B, Schaer JC, Laissue JA. Somatostatin receptor sst1-sst5 expression in normal and neoplastic human tissues using receptor autoradiography with subtype-selective ligands. European Journal of Nuclear Medicine. 2001;**28**(7):836-846. DOI: 10.1007/s002590100541. Erratum in: Eur J Nucl Med 2001 Sep;28(9):1433

[28] Schulz S, Pauli SU, Schulz S, Händel M, Dietzmann K, Firsching R, et al. Immunohistochemical determination of five somatostatin receptors in meningioma reveals frequent overexpression of somatostatin receptor subtype sst2A. Clinical Cancer Research. 2000;**6**(5):1865-1874

[29] Afshar-Oromieh A, Malcher A, Eder M, Eisenhut M, Linhart HG, Hadaschik BA, et al. PET imaging with a [68Ga]gallium-labelled PSMA ligand for the diagnosis of prostate cancer: Biodistribution in humans and first evaluation of tumour lesions. European Journal of Nuclear Medicine and Molecular Imaging. 2013;**40**(4):486-495. DOI: 10.1007/s00259-012-2298-2. Epub 2012 Nov 24. Erratum in: Eur J Nucl Med Mol Imaging. 2013 May;40(5):797-8

[30] Muoio B, Albano D, Dondi F, Bertagna F, Garibotto V, Kunikowska J, et al. Diagnostic accuracy of PET/CT or PET/MRI using PSMA-targeting radiopharmaceuticals in high-grade gliomas: A systematic review and a bivariate meta-analysis. Diagnostics (Basel). 2022;**12**(7):1665. DOI: 10.3390/diagnostics12071665

[31] Al Saffar H, Chen DC, Delgado C, Ingvar J, Hofman MS, Lawrentschuk N, et al. The current landscape of prostate-specific membrane antigen (PSMA) imaging biomarkers for aggressive prostate cancer. Cancers (Basel). 2024;**16**(5):939. DOI: 10.3390/cancers16050939

[32] Sasikumar A, Kashyap R, Joy A, et al. Utility of 68Ga-PSMA-11 PET/CT in imaging of glioma - A pilot study. Clinical Nuclear Medicine. 2018;**43**(9):e304-e309. DOI: 10.1097/RLU.0000000000002175

[33] Jameson JL. Harrison's Endocrinology. 4th ed. New York: McGraw-Hill Education; 2017

[34] Zhang Q, Zang L, Li YJ, Han BY, Gu WJ, Yan WH, et al. Thyrotrophic status in patients with pituitary stalk interruption syndrome. Medicine (Baltimore). 2018;**97**(2):e9084. DOI: 10.1097/MD.0000000000009084

[35] Shimon I, Yan X, Taylor JE, Weiss MH, Culler MD, Melmed S. Somatostatin receptor (SSTR) subtype-selective analogues differentially suppress in vitro growth hormone and prolactin in human pituitary adenomas. Novel potential therapy for functional pituitary tumors. The Journal of Clinical Investigation. 1997;**100**(9):2386-2392. DOI: 10.1172/JCI119779

[36] Taboada GF, Luque RM, Bastos W, Guimarães RF, Marcondes JB, Chimelli LM, et al. Quantitative analysis of somatostatin receptor subtype (SSTR1-5) gene expression levels in somatotropinomas and non-functioning pituitary adenomas. European Journal

of Endocrinology. 2007;**156**(1):65-74. DOI: 10.1530/eje.1.02313

[37] Liu M, Zhai X, Xu T, Duan L, Zhu H, Huo L. Usefulness of ^{68}Ga-FAPI to differentiate sellar-suprasellar lesions. Journal of Nuclear Medicine. 2024;**65**(Supplement 2):241635. Available from: https://jnm.snmjournals.org/content/65/supplement_2/241635

[38] Molitch ME. Pituitary tumours: Pituitary incidentalomas. Best Practice & Research. Clinical Endocrinology & Metabolism. 2009;**23**(5):667-675. DOI: 10.1016/j.beem.2009.05.001

[39] Bajaj S, Krismer F, Palma JA, Wenning GK, Kaufmann H, Poewe W, et al. Diffusion-weighted MRI distinguishes Parkinson disease from the parkinsonian variant of multiple system atrophy: A systematic review and meta-analysis. PLoS One. 2017;**12**(12):e0189897. DOI: 10.1371/journal.pone.0189897

[40] Fanciulli A, Wenning GK. Multiple-system atrophy. The New England Journal of Medicine. 2015;**372**(3):249-263. DOI: 10.1056/NEJMra1311488

[41] Gilman S, Wenning GK, Low PA, Brooks DJ, Mathias CJ, Trojanowski JQ, et al. Second consensus statement on the diagnosis of multiple system atrophy. Neurology. 2008;**71**(9):670-676. DOI: 10.1212/01.wnl.0000324625.00404.15

[42] Watanabe H, Saito Y, Terao S, Ando T, Kachi T, Mukai E, et al. Progression and prognosis in multiple system atrophy: An analysis of 230 Japanese patients. Brain. 2002;**125**(Pt 5):1070-1083. DOI: 10.1093/brain/awf117

[43] Quattrone A, Nicoletti G, Messina D, Fera F, Condino F, Pugliese P, et al. MR imaging index for differentiation of progressive supranuclear palsy from Parkinson disease and the Parkinson variant of multiple system atrophy. Radiology. 2008;**246**(1):214-221. DOI: 10.1148/radiol.2453061703. Epub 2007 Nov 8

[44] Rizzo G, Copetti M, Arcuti S, Martino D, Fontana A, Logroscino G. Accuracy of clinical diagnosis of Parkinson disease: A systematic review and meta-analysis. Neurology. 2016;**86**(6):566-576. DOI: 10.1212/WNL.0000000000002350. Epub 2016 Jan 13

[45] Kraft E, Trenkwalder C, Auer DP. T2-weighted MRI differentiates multiple system atrophy from Parkinson's disease. Neurology. 2002;**59**(8):1265-1267. DOI: 10.1212/01.wnl.0000032757.66992.3c

[46] Bloom GS. Amyloid-β and tau: The trigger and bullet in Alzheimer disease pathogenesis. JAMA Neurology. 2014;**71**(4):505-508. DOI: 10.1001/jamaneurol.2013.5847

[47] 2021 Alzheimer's disease facts and figures. Alzheimer's and Dementia. 2021;**17**(3):327-406. DOI: 10.1002/alz.12328. Epub 2021 Mar 23

[48] Clark CM, Pontecorvo MJ, Beach TG, et al. Cerebral PET with florbetapir compared with neuropathology at autopsy for detection of neuritic amyloid-β plaques: A prospective cohort study [published correction appears in Lancet Neurol. 2012 Aug;11(8):658]. Lancet Neurology. 2012;**11**(8):658-678. DOI: 10.1016/S1474-4422(12)70142-4

[49] Johnson KA, Minoshima S, Bohnen NI, et al. Appropriate use criteria for amyloid PET: A report of the Amyloid Imaging Task Force, the Society of Nuclear Medicine and Molecular Imaging, and the Alzheimer's

Association. Alzheimer's and Dementia. 2013;**9**(1):e-16. DOI: 10.1016/j.jalz.2013.01.002

[50] Ossenkoppele R, Pichet Binette A, Groot C, et al. Amyloid and tau PET-positive cognitively unimpaired individuals are at high risk for future cognitive decline. Nature Medicine. 2022;**28**(11):2381-2387. DOI: 10.1038/s41591-022-02049-x

[51] Jessen F, Amariglio RE, van Boxtel M, et al. A conceptual framework for research on subjective cognitive decline in preclinical Alzheimer's disease. Alzheimer's and Dementia. 2014;**10**(6):844-852. DOI: 10.1016/j.jalz.2014.01.001

[52] Schöll M, Lockhart SN, Schonhaut DR, et al. PET imaging of tau deposition in the aging human brain. Neuron. 2016;**89**(5):971-982. DOI: 10.1016/j.neuron.2016.01.028

[53] Jagust WJ, Landau SM, Koeppe RA, et al. The Alzheimer's disease neuroimaging initiative 2 PET core: 2015. Alzheimer's and Dementia. 2015;**11**(7):757-771. DOI: 10.1016/j.jalz.2015.05.001

[54] Palmqvist S, Janelidze S, Quiroz YT, et al. Discriminative accuracy of plasma phospho-tau217 for Alzheimer disease vs other neurodegenerative disorders. JAMA. 2020;**324**(8):772-781. DOI: 10.1001/jama.2020.12134

[55] Doraiswamy PM, Sperling RA, Coleman RE, et al. Amyloid-β assessed by florbetapir F 18 PET and 18-month cognitive decline: A multicenter study. Neurology. 2012;**79**(16):1636-1644. DOI: 10.1212/WNL.0b013e3182661f74

Section 3

Interventional Neuroimaging and Neuronavigation

Chapter 5

Interventional Neuroimaging: Techniques, Applications, and Future Directions

Naheed Akhter, Sadia Sana, Yasmin Mushtaq, Mamoona Tariq and Maryam Afzaal

Abstract

Interventional neuroimaging represents a transformative approach to understanding, diagnosing, and treating neurodegenerative diseases. This chapter explores the foundational principles of bio-imaging about neurodegenerative conditions such as Alzheimer's Disease, Parkinson's Disease, and Huntington's Disease. It highlights the role of advanced imaging modalities, including structural, functional, molecular, and hybrid techniques, in detecting disease-specific biomarkers, monitoring progression, and guiding therapeutic strategies. The integration of cutting-edge technologies like artificial intelligence, ultrahigh-field imaging, and multimodal approaches is discussed as a pivotal factor in shaping the future of neuroimaging. Furthermore, the chapter delves into the applications of neuroimaging for early diagnosis, disease monitoring, and personalized medicine. Emphasizing current advancements and future directions, this chapter underscores the critical role of neuroimaging in revolutionizing neuroscience and clinical practice.

Keywords: neuroimaging, interventional neuroimaging, neurodegenerative diseases, biomarkers, structural imaging, functional imaging, magnetic resonance imaging (MRI), positron emission tomography (PET), diffusion tensor imaging (DTI)

1. Introduction

1.1 Bio-imaging and neurodegenerative disease

Millions of individuals worldwide struggle with neurodegenerative disorders (NDs), making them one of the most significant health challenges in modern society [1]. Although metabolic or toxic diseases cause selective static neuronal loss, neurodegenerative disorders lead to the gradual disappearance of selectively sensitive groups of neurons [2]. These disorders result in a continuous decline in neuronal function, ultimately leading to brain shrinkage.

Age is the most significant risk factor for the development of all NDs; however, recent research suggests that both genetic and environmental factors play an equally important role in determining an individual's susceptibility to these disorders.

Furthermore, even though certain genes responsible for NDs are expressed in all individuals, on a global scale, the annual incidence of NDs is generally reported to be between 10 and 15 per 100,000 individuals [3, 4]. The diverse clinical symptoms of NDs make diagnosis challenging, often requiring a neuropathological examination, which is typically performed postmortem [5].

In neurodegenerative disorders, harmful processes such as protein accumulation, neuronal loss, and inflammation impact brain structure and function [6]. Advanced imaging techniques such as MRI and PET allow researchers to document these alterations in living subjects, enabling early detection, disease monitoring, and the development of targeted treatment strategies.

1.2 Natural products as therapeutic agents for neurodegenerative disorders

Traditional medicines have long played a crucial role in meeting basic healthcare needs, particularly in developing countries, and remain fundamental to public health systems [7]. Research indicates that natural substances are a significant source of pharmacological leads and bioactive compounds [8, 9]. Consequently, the therapeutic potential of natural derivatives continues to be explored in modern medicine. Studies have demonstrated that natural derivatives offer a promising approach to discovering innovative and biologically active drugs [10].

For thousands of years, people have used medicinal herbs to treat various illnesses and improve overall well-being [11]. In recent years, research on natural products and their bioactive components has expanded significantly, recognizing their potential as superior biological and therapeutic agents for NDs. Natural substances hold great promise for both the treatment and prevention of these disorders. However, clinical reservations persist due to insufficient scientific evidence supporting their efficacy and patient safety [12].

The value of plant-based natural derivatives is evident, as many of the currently available medications for NDs originate from plant sources. For example, plants are the primary source of opioids, alkaloids, and anticholinesterase compounds such as galantamine, physostigmine, and neostigmine [9].

1.3 The pathophysiological mechanism of neurodegeneration

1.3.1 Oxidative stress and inflammation

In 1985, oxidative stress was first used. Hydrogen peroxide (H_2O_2), hydroxyl radicals (OH), superoxide (O^{2-}), lipids radicals, and nitric oxide (NO) are examples of reactive oxygen species, a class of highly reactive, short-half-life compounds generated from oxygen [13, 14]. Both endogenous and exogenous external generation of ROS are possible. Endogenous sources include enzymes that produce ROS in or outside mitochondria, while exogenous sources include the metabolism of ambient substances, medications, and ionizing radiation [15]. In healthy cells, electrons leaving mitochondrial transport chains generate more than 90% of reactive oxygen species and enzymes produce the remaining 10% [16, 17]. As a result of higher oxygen consumption, high levels of ROS are produced in the brain, which influence biomolecules such as RNA, proteins, lipids, DNA, and processes including peroxidation and oxidation [13]. Protein and lipid oxidation is more vital than DNA oxidation in complex organisms like humans, especially in NDDs, where oxidized proteins can become hazardous (**Figure 1**) [17].

DOI: http://dx.doi.org/10.5772/intechopen.1009438

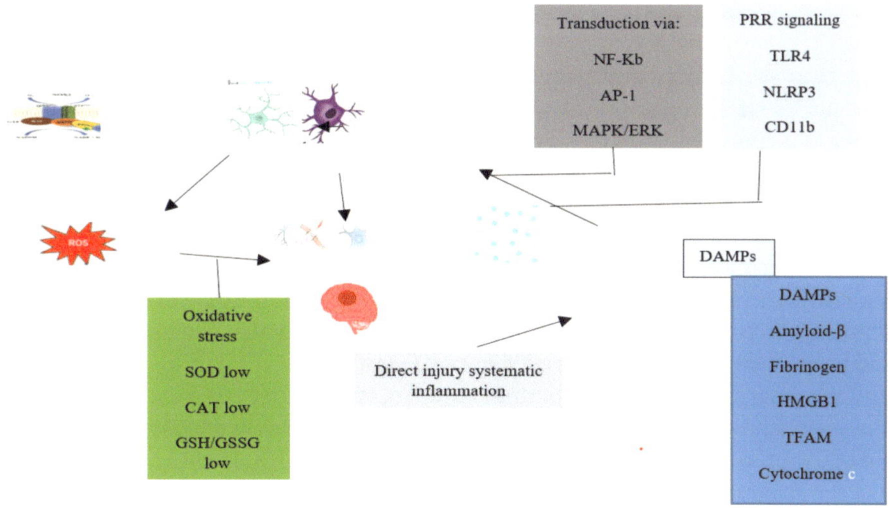

Figure 1.
Pathophysiological pathways in neurodegenerative diseases: Oxidative stress, DAMPs, and PRR signaling.

1.3.2 Mitochondrial dysfunction

Since neurons demand a lot of energy and oxygen, they are prone to injury and may be the source of several neurodegenerative diseases [18]. Because mitochondria fuel neurons, any modifications to the structure of the mitochondria can affect ATP biosynthesis and possibly cause NDs [19, 20]. Crucial cell organelles, via modifying their dynamics in a spatiotemporal manner, mitochondria play a significant part in the generation of cellular energy [21, 22]. Despite producing ATP, mitochondria also manage oxidative stress, maintain Ca2+ homeostasis, and cellular signaling metabolism (**Figure 2**) [20, 23].

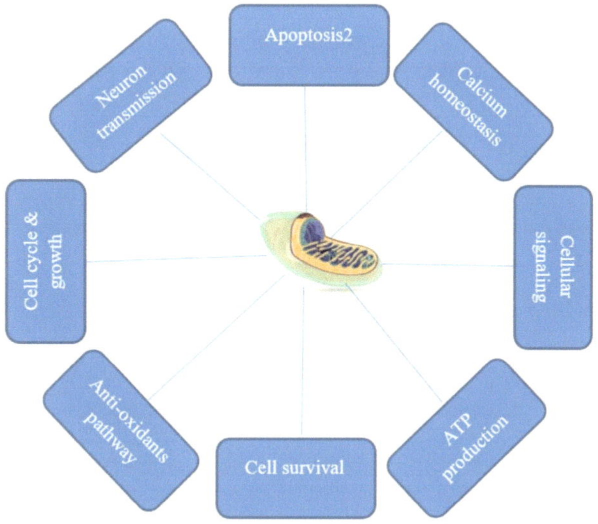

Figure 2.
Key roles of mitochondria in cellular function and homeostasis.

1.3.3 Mitochondrial dysfunction in AD, PD

The most widespread neurodegenerative illness is AD, which affects 1–3% of people and 10–15% of persons over 65 [24]. Dementia is a condition characterized by memory and executive dysfunction, affecting daily life, but can also involve a typical presentation affecting language, visual, or executive function [25]. Some researchers have even put out the mitochondrial cascade theory, which suggests a number of mechanisms including mitochondrial dysfunction. In accordance with the amyloid hypothesis, the disease's primary cause is believed to be the aberrant accumulation of amyloid plaques outside the cells of specific brain regions. According to this viewpoint, the participation of particular cellular components, such as mitochondria, would be considered a secondary occurrence (**Figure 3**).

In Alzheimer's disease, mitochondrial failure occurs. Numerous data, such as decreased glucose and oxygen consumption in the patient's brain and altered DNA shape, imply faulty mitochondrial functioning and impairment of respiratory chain disorder. It has been suggested that mitochondrial failure is reciprocally related to the buildup of intracellular tau protein and extracellular Aβ, two of the most common neuropathological failures in AD. The illness has been linked to changes in mitochondrial DNA.

The second most common neurodegenerative disorder is PD. Under a microscope, PD is identified by the intracellular protein clusters, called Lewy bodies, that are primarily made up of alpha-synuclein (**Figure 4**) [26].

PD is linked with mitochondrial dysfunction. Clinical and neuropathological Parkinsonian characteristics are brought on by mitochondrial inhibitors (MPTP and rotenone) and defective respiratory chain activity, particularly complex 1. Alpha-synuclein buildup inside cells is reciprocally associated with mitochondrial dysfunction. There have been reports of mitochondrial DNA A alteration such as point mutation, depletion, deletion, and poor maintenance.

1.3.4 Misfolded protein's role

1.3.4.1 Protein's misfolding mechanism and intermediate

Misfolding is an incorrect folding process that results in a protein with a different conformation than its initial fold. There are several causes for protein misfolding [27, 28]:

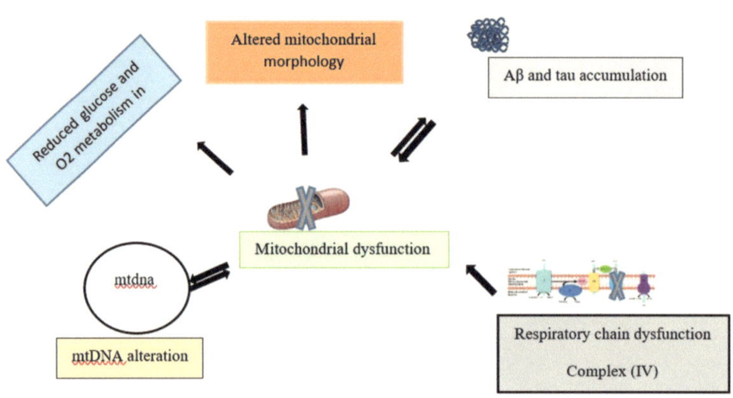

Figure 3.
Mitochondrial functions in cellular processes: A central role in homeostasis and survival.

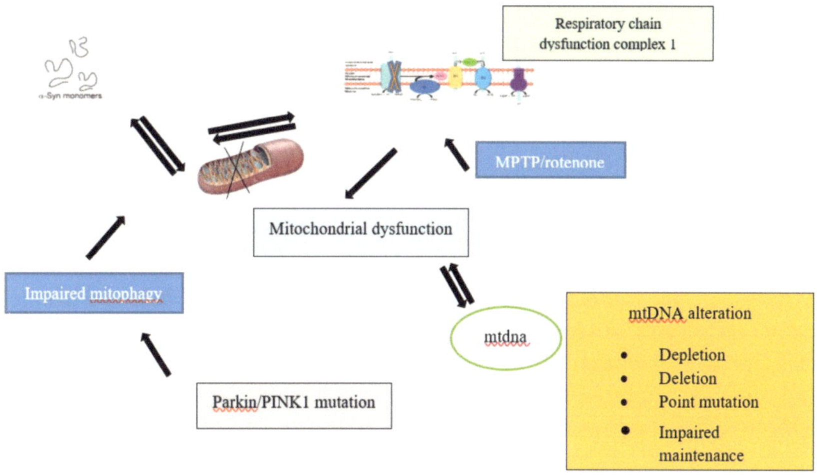

Figure 4.
Mitochondrial roles in cellular function and regulation.

(1) somatic gene sequence mutation that produces proteins incapable of adjusting to their natural folding; (2) transcriptional and translational errors that result in the production of misfolded proteins that cannot fold properly; (3) malfunctions in the folding and chaperone machinery; (4) errors in post-translational modification or protein trafficking; (5) structural changes brought on by environmental changes; or (6) seeding and cross-seeding mechanisms that induce protein misfolding (**Figure 5**).

1.3.4.2 Biomarkers and diagnosis of neurodegenerative disease

Neurodegenerative disease diagnosis is a difficult process. Clinical evaluation is the primary foundation of the diagnostic procedure. Although functional imaging is frequently used to rule out other diagnoses, an increasing amount of research suggested that imaging could assist in identifying dementia and parkinsonism early because it may have a higher specificity for neurodegenerative diseases [29].

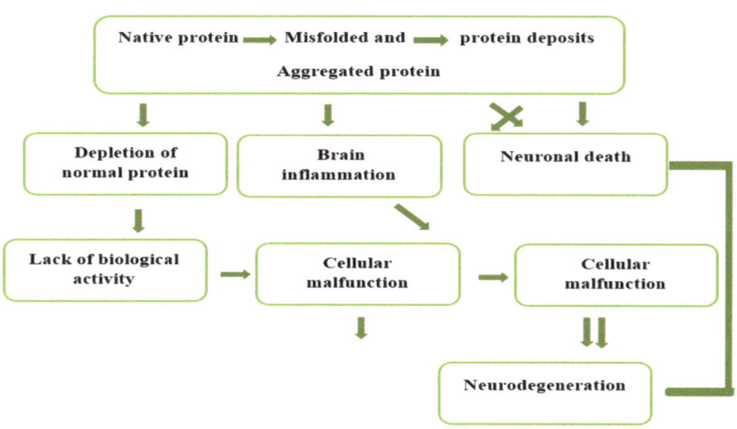

Figure 5.
Mitochondrial functions in cellular processes.

In addition to diagnosing NDs, protein biomarkers may be useful in monitoring the progression of dementia in patients suffering from cognitive impairments and forecasting future cognitive decline in healthy people. Additionally, it is possible to use some markers to evaluate the effectiveness of treatment, allowing for the creation of novel therapeutic approaches [30]. Blood-based biomarkers are advantageous since they are inexpensive, easy to use, and require less invasiveness during blood collection. For many years, plasma biomarkers were measured using several analytical platforms. For CSF assay, ELISA was first created and is among the most widely used methods. However, it turned out that there were methodological problems with plasma that had a big impact on the ELISA's performance. One of the earliest technologies to replace ELISA was Multiple Analyte Profiling (xMAP technology), which optimizes the overall workflow for biomarker analysis and requires less material by detecting multiple analytes simultaneously. Since both systems have shown increased sensitivity in detecting lower quantities of biomarkers, mesoscale discovery (MSD) and electrochemiluminescence (ECL) are becoming more and more popular as stand-ins for conventional ELISA and xMAP technologies. To figure out their diagnostic qualities, additional prospective research is required. The recently invented single molecular assay (SIMOA) technology, which enables the detection of incredibly minute amounts, improves sensitivity and excellent diagnostic accuracy. SIMOA technique is based on the simultaneous counting of simulated capture microbeads and single molecule arrays. Clinically speaking, fully automated technologies like the SIMOA or ECL appear to be the most dependable approach for the quantitative evaluation of blood biomarkers [31].

1.4 Bio-imaging

1.4.1 Clinical signs and trials for neurodegenerative disease

The pathophysiology of neurodegenerative disease is better understood thanks to recent developments in neurobiology, which have also made it possible to design medication-based treatments. However, currently available therapeutic medications mostly aid in maintaining a patient's condition and keeping them from getting worse rather than stopping the evolution of the disease. Choline esterase activity inhibition may alleviate cognitive and memory defects by raising acetylcholine levels. A small amount of AD was prevented by a few cholinesterase inhibitors, including rivastigmine, galantamine, donepezil, and huperzine A [32]. Furthermore, neuronal dysfunction in AD is caused by aberrant glutamate levels. Consequently, medications that stop the overstimulation of the NMDA receptor, such as namzaric and memantine, have been beneficial for AD patients [33]. Another therapy for AD is Axona (caprylidene), a medication that raises the concentration of ketone bodies, which subsequently give neurons energy [34]. Bradykinesia, stiffness, Tremor, and postural instability are hallmarks of PD. PD is currently related to medication and surgery. Levodopa is showing promise as a medication to treat bradykinesia-related PD symptoms [35]. In the early stages of PD, dopamine agonists like ropinirole are useful medications [36].

Neuroimaging techniques like positron emission tomography (PET) and magnetic resonance imaging (MRI) have provided essential insights into neurodegenerative diseases such as Alzheimer's and Parkinson's. PET scans using tracers such as fluorodeoxyglucose (FDG) reveal metabolic activity in the brain, allowing for early detection of AD. Structural MRI aids in identifying hippocampal atrophy, a hallmark of AD, while functional MRI (fMRI) has been used to study disrupted neural networks in PD. Such advancements enable the identification of disease progression and efficacy of interventions during clinical trials.

1.4.2 Bioactive compounds

Each day, there is a remarkable surge in concern about bioactive substances, which has also invoked the interest of scholars to pay attention to the bioactive compounds in food resources like fruit, vegetables, flavors, herbs, and spices being used in daily life. Higher interest was elevated and led to the novel research region to discover useful disease-oriented research of Tannins, Flavonoids, Alkaloids, and also phenolic complexes. Every plant and its parts possess these compounds, their metabolites, or derivatives, or originate products like plant-based food (fruits and vegetables) in small or very small proportions. These major natural resources have indifferent to most often beneficial meta-immunological effects in the body to maintain and promote healthy health. Oftentimes, the term bioactive substances is used to refer to auxiliary metabolites that are not vital to the life of the plant but are extremely useful in cases of competition, protection, attraction, and communication. Some of such compounds can be referred to as "auxiliary plant metabolites," meaning they have therapeutic activity in humans and animals. Bioactive substances provide therapeutic effects by interacting with biological systems and regulating processes such as immunological response, inflammation, and cell proliferation. They can help to cure infection, cancer, and chronic disorders by altering certain biological targets. Neuroimaging techniques like PET and fMRI are vital for assessing the therapeutic effects of bioactive agents, enabling real-time monitoring of brain activity, receptor binding, and metabolic changes in preclinical and clinical studies.

1.4.3 Bioflavonoids

Bioflavonoids are the frequent and widespread phenols in the landscape. In general, flavonoids are believed to contribute to the pigment and aroma of foods. Apart from this broad classification, this group also plays a role in preventing fat oxidation, maintaining food quality, and preserving the quantity of enzymes and vitamins [37]. Bioflavonoids can be divided into six subclasses, including anthocyanins, flavonols, flavanols, and flavanones (**Figure 6**).

Neurological conditions can be characterized as the chronic primary dysfunction of a defined populace of neurons, resulting in sensory-motor dysfunction and cognitive deterioration. There are multiple signaling mechanisms involved in neurological conditions, which include inflammation, free radical damage, and cell death. In this regard, polyphenols are capable of directly neutralizing the free radical species, with the suppression of the so-called "pro-oxidant" enzymes, the stimulation of inherent antioxidant enzymes [38], or interference with apoptotic pathways [39]. Polyphenols work in a way through a mechanism of inhibiting the genetic damage produced by H_2O_2 and metals. DNA damage due to Au-iron-mediated hydroxyl radical is the principal feature of cell death under conditions of oxidative pressure for mutually prokaryotic and eukaryotic cells. The molecular mechanism of neuroprotection includes one important cellular signaling pathway, which is the mitochondrial apoptosis cascade that is regarded as the stability of Bcl-2 and Bax, the two types of proteins. Phytochemical neuroprotection may be attained by manifestation of the anti-apoptotic Bcl-2 that will deter apoptosis [40]. In the event of bioactive phenolic

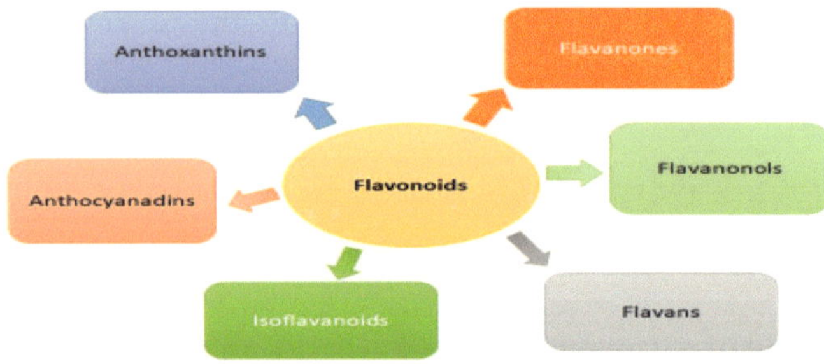

Figure 6.
Classification of flavonoids.

amalgams, the beneficial health impact is, therefore, clinically delineated by the accessibility and assimilation rate. These properties can be "fine-tuned" via the effects of other nutrients present in the diet and by the act of enzymatic processes within the intestine and liver. In people's bodies, polyphenols are frequently acknowledged as xenobiotics. Their passive diffusion across the mucosa of the gut after ingestion can also be enhanced after certain biochemical transformations such as methylation, sulfonation, and glucuronidation [41]. Polyphenols are active in neuroprotection primarily by acting on neuroscience and secondarily through the interactions with gut microbiota and its byproducts.

1.4.4 Study on oxidative stress and polyphenols

Oxygen-reactive species-related oxidative damage is determined by excess production and poor elimination capabilities within the cells. ROS is an oxymoron intended for the cells. They are generated during normal digestion as intermediates in numerous physiological processes and, when present at physiological levels, they regulate redox balance within the cell. However, any disparity between their synthesis and the capacity of the cell to monitor and constrain their utilization may impact the cell structure and functionality, potentially leading to cell destruction and eventual death [42].

1.4.5 Antioxidant plant

The negative properties of ROS can be neutralized by the effects of antioxidants. They are described as chemicals capable of preventing the corrosion of any molecule including at a very low deliberation. They exercise their function by preventing or stopping free radical reactions and, therefore, reducing the rates of injury to cells. Overwhelmingly, it is agreed that neurodegeneration development is accompanied by stresses that define the gravity of an injury in the cell. Surprisingly, oxidative stress can produce significant damage on a deeper biological level. The lack of proper redox control defines an excess of ROS associated with the constant promotion of cellular impairment with neurodegenerative features; this is essential in neurodegenerative ailments. The production of a large amount of ROS in nervous tissue is attributed to excitatory amino acids and neurotransmitters [43]. Consequently, nerve cells require free radical scavengers to neutralize and eliminate ROS. The body's defense against ROS consists of an enzyme-based antioxidant system. The antioxidant proteins lowered the lipid hydroperoxide; therefore, they

DOI: http://dx.doi.org/10.5772/intechopen.1009438

should play major roles in minimizing lipid oxidation and the preservation of stability, fluidity, and performance of the membrane.

Non-enzymatic oxidants are the radicals that occur naturally in the plant. It was observed that polyphenols are the most potent ROS scavengers capable of regulating cellular ROS through the activation of antioxidant signaling pathways [44].

1.4.6 Phenolic acids and their function

Phenolic acids show their antioxidant exploitation by capturing free radicals [45]. It was, however, reported that the antioxidant effect of phenolic triterpenes is ascribed to the actions of lipid free radicals and low-density lipoprotein oxidation. Antioxidant properties of volatile oils partially depend on the phenolic compounds, which are reacted with peroxyl radicals. The most populous class of polyphenolic compounds in plants is flavonoids because of their potential metal-fixing and free radical inhibitors [46]. In contrast, there is interaction between stilbenes and hydroxyl radicals in that stilbenes consume them.

Other polyphenols in foods in addition to flavonoids are known to possess antioxidant activity. Of these, curcumin from Curcuma longa acts to inhibit the peroxidation of lipids by removing hydrogen peroxide and hydroxyl (OH) radicals [47].

1.4.7 Molecular mechanisms through which polyphenols confer neuroprotection

While cells contain a broad spectrum of antioxidants, body cells and organs are even more liable to oxidative damage than others, most likely due to increased levels of oxygen ingestion and the resultant production of ROS. Several considerations indicate that the brain is especially liable tissue to the belongings of oxidative stress [48] and oxidative stress has been occupied in the genesis of a widespread variety of clinical ailments and the aging process. Hyperopic stress is reported to be higher in many age-induced degenerative ailments, counting some genetic diseases of neurodegeneration diseases (AD, PD, MS) [49]. This is the reason why neurons are extremely prone to oxidative damage like other post-mitotic cells, as they cannot be replenished. Similarly, the ability of cells to respond to oxidative protein impairment also appears to decrease with age [50].

Polyphenols such as resveratrol and curcumin possess the ability to defend against neurodegenerative disorders by triggering protein kinase-mediated signaling pathways, the major neuroprotective pathway against internal and external influences, including ROS-induced oxidative stress [51]. Through the binding to these bioactive molecules, Keap1 and Nrf2 complex is disrupted, allowing Nrf2 to translocate to the nucleus, bind to adenylyl and uridylyl abundant response elements (AREs), and activate the antioxidant appearance of HO-1 [51]. The phytochemical polyphenols also increase neurotrophic growth factors with a central responsibility in sustaining the health of neurons. They include, for instance, BDNF, which plays a central role in erudition and memory. Nerve growth factor (NGF) is important in the existence of nerves within the brain and the Glial cell-line-derivative neurotrophic factor (GDNF), which is involved in cellular survival and synaptic flexibility. In the current study, genistein and quercetin were found to promote NGF-mediated neurite extension. Resveratrol also promotes the production of GDNF and BDNF, thereby safeguarding cells from neurotoxicity [52]. The neuroprotective effects of polyphenols are exerted through preclinical signaling cascades, which, in cells, maintain pathways involved in post-transcription, post-translation, production, development, and existence that includes the "PI3K/Akt-ERK signaling pathways".

1.4.8 Role of polyphenol in neurodegenerative diseases

Despite the clinical signs of the neurodegenerative diseases described above are quite diverse, these diseases have similar molecular pathogenesis mechanisms. The authors affirmed that in Alzheimer's disease, Parkinson's disease, and dementia, the breakdown of the roles of the neurovascular units occurs due to inflammation and oxidative stress. ROS are capable of engaging with variegated neuronal signaling systems, including protein kinase and lipid kinase signaling transduction [53].

1.5 Alzheimer's disease (AD)

Neurodegenerative disorder Alzheimer's disease (AD) affects generally all dementia diseases and implies progressive destruction of neurons [54]. Amyloid, which is composed of amyloid beta (Aβ) protein, forms extracellular amyloid plaques and neurofibrillary tangles [55], which previously caused a predisposed gradual decline in the general structure of the brain and the eventual loss of intellect function. Increased concentrations of Aβ peptides and ROS enhance inhibitory cell death in AD and downregulate phosphatidylinositol-4,5-bisphosphate 3-kinase (PI3K)/protein kinase B (Akt) pathway. Akt inactivation controls diverse apoptotic signaling molecules. These receptors affect amyloid genesis in the brain region and specifically in AD; curcumin possesses the anti-amyloid genic effect and influences the mitogen-activated protein kinase (MAPK) and phosphatidylinositol-3-kinase (PI3K) pathways. Furthermore, turmeric extract curcumin is capable of preventing the reduction in BDNF in mice injected with Amyloid beta peptide through altering phosphatidylinositol 3-kinase (PI3K)/protein kinase B (Akt)/glycogen synthase kinase-3 β (GSK3β) pathway that led to intellectual enhancement.

In more recent studies, the antioxidant activity of resveratrol produces a positive impact on the protection of memory deterioration in AD. In cells, some studies showed that polyphenol compound resveratrol reduces Aβ-stimulated ROS production and cell death. Studies documented suggested that resveratrol has neuroprotective effects by regulating the phosphatidylinositol-3-kinase (PI3K)/protein kinase B (Akt) signaling pathway. In the brain, SIRT is neuroprotective and protects neurons against neurodegeneration by acetylating a variety of transcription influences and stress-resistance proteins. In particular, this ability is associated with PGC-1α deacetylation, sharing active PPAR-γ, and Bcl-2 upregulation, protecting against mitochondria damage. In animal studies, EGCG was reported to be active toward AD being capable of reducing cognitive loss and Aβ peptides while enhancing proteins associated with synaptic plasticity [56]. EGCG averts Neuronal apoptosis from neurotoxic processes that are due to the inhibition of BACE. Experiments described the neuroprotective effects of quercetin in Aβ toxicity, showing a correlation between this polyphenol and increased cell viability as well as decreased oxidative stress neurons. Quercetin appears to prevent the formation of Aβ plaque and the development of neurofibrillary tangle, perhaps through enhancing Apolipoprotein E, which plays a crucial role in Aβ clearance [57]. Flavonoids contributed to the diminishment of the Beta-amyloid fibrils with the enhancement of cognitive functions.

1.6 Parkinson's disease (PD)

Parkinson's disease is a progressive neural disease defined by the progressive degeneration of dopamine-producing neurons in the substantia nigra, which defines clinical motor signs including rigidity, bradykinesia, and tremor [58]. There is still high acceptance of the oxidative stress hypothesis in attributing the advanced fading of dopaminergic neurons in the substantia nigra of PD patients. ROS found in microglia through NADPH oxidase stimulate PKc delta and ERK1/2, which activate the genes responsible for apoptosis [59]. Molecular mechanism recommends that flavonoid quercetin has the aptitude to rejuvenate damaged mitochondrial electron transport. It was also concluded from laboratory and animal models that Curcumin alleviates oxidative stress in toxin-induced Parkinson's disease by reducing apoptosis through signaling pathway, with Nrf2 transcription enhancing antioxidant enzyme activation [60]. Studies also noted that curcumin in PD beats the suppression of the enzyme tyrosine hydroxylase, which is recognized to be a crucial factor responsible for the progress of PD [61]. Current research on curcumin demonstrated that it has ameliorative belongings in PD by preventing oxidative stress through the reduction of ROS, tumor necrosis factor alpha, and interleukin-6, as well as the upregulation of Glutathione-coupled (GSH) system. On the other hand, in PD, curcumin acts as both an antioxidant and an anti-inflammatory agent, additionally decreasing the formation of TNF-α and Interleukin-6 (IL-6). The protective role of turmeric extract-curcumin on PD pathogenesis can also be associated with the capacity to lower TLR4 as well as its subsequent signaling molecules including NF-κB IRF3 and MyD88 [62].

In all these cases, the PD-affected pathway indicates that Resveratrol appears to be a direct modulator. In vitro experiments provide evidence that this molecule still antagonizes rotenone's effect on this auto phagocytic dysfunction and encourages α-synuclein degradation [63]. Another experiment indicated that resveratrol exerts a protective action through the modulation of the phosphatidylinositol 3-kinase (PI3K)/protein kinase B (Akt)/glycogen synthase kinase-3 β (GSK3β) pathway or the downregulation of apoptosis by antioxidant enzymes. Furthermore, it has been evidenced that quercetin inhibits glutathione and, at the same time, stimulates the activity of both catalase CAT and SOD. In PD, neuron protection of EGCG through AMPK stimulation and enhancement of dopaminergic neuronal required mitochondrial biogenesis.

1.7 Huntington's disease (HD) and neurocognitive disorders

Huntington's disease (HD) and neurocognitive disorders are two other neurodegenerative disorders that are also totally compromised with cognition apart from AD and PD. The function of polyphenols in preventing is not searched so actively in these NDs-AD and PD. Huntington's disease is a dominant autosomal disorder that presents clinical features that are due to neuron death and atrophy in the neostriatum and cortex. The pathogenic allele is an increased number of CAG repeats (>36) in the coding sequence, encoding a polyglutamine region in the N-terminal end of the huntingtin protein, which is ubiquitously expressed, though its function is still unknown [64]. Mutated Huntington's is stated not only in brain neurons but also in gastrointestinal neurons [65]. Huntington's disorder has also been linked with mitochondrial impairment and oxidative damage as potential ailment processes. HD cellular models were linked to decreased mitochondrial function with mitochondrial membrane potential and respiration becoming deregulated.

The antioxidant and neuroprotective action of flavonoid curcumin has been described only lately, in a transgenic animal model of HD. This research affirmed that curcumin safeguarded the brain against neuropathological and phenotypic changes that are proportional to the illness. However, it has been described that resveratrol in HD upregulates genes connected to mitochondrial biogenesis. In the present case, resveratrol in HD appears to influence SIRT in some form. In studying mouse models of HD, resveratrol was demonstrated to considerably increase the expression of mitochondrial genes and improve mitochondrial function. This activity was followed by the assessment and enhancement of motor function in HD transgenic mouse models. However, quercetin was able to prevent mitochondrial oxidative damage in HD. This effect results in the enhancement of motor proficiency and coordination as indicated in the drug-induced HD model. Actually, in core lesions, less increase in astrocyte count and a reduction in microglial proliferation with decreased neuro-inflammatory response were seen, for which the sickle cell mice showed improvement in neurological symptoms [66].

Resveratrol was neuroprotective in neurocognitive disorders since it reduced cell death in the brain part hippocampus and recovered reference memory [67]. In the animal model of vascular dementia, cognitive performance improved and oxidative damage levels were revered due to the deficiency of BDNF [68]. Quercetin ameliorates cognitive deficiency and energy metabolism in the peptide model of dementia by directly and indirectly neutralizing radical species and inhibiting a range of oxidases [69]. The neuroprotective potential of bioactive substances is significant, with interventional neuroimaging techniques like PET, fMRI, and DTI allowing for detailed real-timing imaging of how these substances interact with the brain and influence neural activity. By visualization, these effects of neuroimaging exert their therapeutic benefits.

2. Neuroimaging techniques for neurodegenerative disease

Interventional neuroimaging has revolutionized our understanding and management of neurodegenerative diseases by enabling visualization of intricate brain structures and functions. These advancements have paved the way for targeted therapies and precision medicine, fostering hope for mitigating disease progression [70].

Misfolded proteins, such as amyloid-β in Alzheimer's Disease (AD) and α-synuclein in Parkinson's Disease (PD), play critical roles in neurodegenerative pathology. Advanced neuroimaging modalities like positron emission tomography (PET) and magnetic resonance imaging (MRI) facilitate the visualization of these pathogenic proteins, aiding in early diagnosis and therapeutic monitoring [71].

Neuroimaging techniques are integral to clinical trials, helping to stratify patients, monitor disease progression, and evaluate therapeutic efficacy. For instance, functional MRI (fMRI) captures brain activity patterns, providing insights into cognitive decline in conditions like AD and Huntington's Disease (HD).

Emerging neuroimaging approaches facilitate the evaluation of bioactive compounds targeting neurodegenerative diseases. Techniques like single-photon emission computed tomography (SPECT) enable real-time tracking of pharmacokinetics and pharmacodynamics, ensuring therapeutic precision.

Neuroimaging modalities like PET scans with amyloid and tau tracers are pivotal in diagnosing and staging AD. Moreover, diffusion tensor imaging (DTI) elucidates

DOI: http://dx.doi.org/10.5772/intechopen.1009438

white matter integrity, revealing early microstructural changes associated with the disease [72].

Advanced imaging techniques, such as DaT-SPECT, assess dopaminergic neuron loss in PD, facilitating early and differential diagnosis. Additionally, ultrahigh-field MRI offers unprecedented resolution for visualizing brainstem nuclei, aiding in understanding disease mechanisms [73].

Quantitative MRI metrics, such as volumetric analyses, are instrumental in monitoring neurodegeneration in HD. Functional imaging, including resting-state fMRI, uncovers connectivity alterations in neurocognitive disorders, offering biomarkers for disease progression.

Neuroimaging plays a pivotal role in understanding the progression of brain degenerative diseases, offering a window into the pathophysiology of disorders like multiple sclerosis (MS), frontotemporal dementia (FTD), and amyotrophic lateral sclerosis (ALS). Techniques like volumetric MRI provide detailed assessments of cortical thinning and subcortical atrophy, while advanced diffusion imaging reveals microstructural disruptions in white matter tracts. Additionally, MR spectroscopy uncovers metabolic abnormalities in brain tissues, complementing functional imaging modalities in tracking neural dysfunction and compensatory mechanisms. These insights facilitate timely diagnosis, guide therapeutic interventions, and improve the accuracy of prognostic models.

2.1 Structural neuroimaging

Structural imaging techniques, such as MRI and computed tomography (CT), provide high-resolution anatomical details. These methods are indispensable for detecting structural abnormalities like brain atrophy, vascular lesions, and hydrocephalus in neurodegenerative conditions [74].

MRI is one of the most widely used techniques in neurodegenerative disease research. It enables detailed visualization of brain atrophy, which is a hallmark of diseases such as Alzheimer's Disease (AD), Parkinson's Disease (PD), and Huntington's Disease (HD). Quantitative MRI techniques, such as voxel-based morphometry (VBM) and cortical thickness analysis, provide high-resolution data to monitor disease progression.

Computed Tomography (CT): Although less commonly used than MRI, CT scans can still provide useful information in acute changes or when MRI is contraindicated. It helps assess structural changes in the brain, particularly in vascular dementia [75].

2.2 Functional neuroimaging

Functional neuroimaging, including fMRI and PET, maps neural activity by detecting changes in blood flow or metabolic processes. These techniques offer insights into brain networks involved in cognition, emotion, and motor control, facilitating early disease detection [76].

Diffusion Tensor Imaging is an advanced MRI technique that maps the brain's white matter tracts, which are often disrupted in neurodegenerative diseases. This imaging modality is particularly useful for detecting early changes in diseases such as AD, where disruptions in the hippocampal and cortical networks can be seen before more obvious atrophy occurs [74].

Magnetic Resonance Spectroscopy (MRS) allows for the measurement of metabolites within the brain, such as N-acetyl aspartate (NAA), choline, and creatine.

Alterations in these metabolites can be indicative of neuronal loss or dysfunction, which is relevant in understanding diseases like AD, PD, and HD.

PET imaging with radiotracers such as fluorodeoxyglucose (FDG) is valuable for detecting early metabolic changes in neurodegenerative diseases. It has also been used to evaluate amyloid and tau deposition in AD. PET imaging helps identify dopaminergic dysfunction in PD, which is crucial for early diagnosis and treatment planning.

Single-Photon Emission Computed Tomography (SPECT): SPECT offers functional imaging similar to PET, though with a lower spatial resolution. It is particularly useful in evaluating brain perfusion and dopamine transporter activity, which is key in diseases like PD and HD [77].

2.3 Molecular imaging

Molecular imaging employs radiolabeled tracers to visualize biochemical processes in vivo. For example, PET imaging with fluorodeoxyglucose (FDG) highlights metabolic deficits in neurodegenerative diseases, while novel tracers target specific pathological proteins [78].

2.4 Hybrid imaging

Hybrid imaging modalities, such as PET/MRI and PET/CT, combine the strengths of structural and functional imaging. These approaches enhance diagnostic accuracy and provide comprehensive assessments of neurodegenerative diseases [79].

3. Applications of neuroimaging in neurodegenerative diseases

3.1 Early diagnosis

Pre-symptomatic Detection: Neuroimaging, particularly structural MRI and PET, is becoming increasingly valuable in detecting subtle brain changes before clinical symptoms appear. For instance, the use of amyloid PET scans has revolutionized early diagnosis in AD, allowing for the detection of amyloid plaques years before cognitive decline becomes noticeable.

Differential Diagnosis: Neuroimaging is crucial in differentiating between various neurodegenerative diseases, as many share overlapping symptoms. For example, MRI is used to distinguish between AD and frontotemporal dementia (FTD) by identifying specific patterns of atrophy. PET imaging with tau and amyloid tracers can also differentiate AD from other dementias [80].

3.2 Disease monitoring

Quantitative Imaging Biomarkers: The use of quantitative metrics obtained from MRI, PET, and SPECT scans enables clinicians to monitor disease progression over time. For example, volumetric changes in the hippocampus, measured through MRI, are considered a key biomarker of AD progression [73].

Functional Imaging for Symptom Correlation: Functional imaging (PET, SPECT) can be used to correlate brain activity with clinical symptoms, improving our understanding of the relationship between cognitive decline and functional brain alterations.

3.3 Treatment planning and response assessment

Monitoring Therapeutic Interventions: Neuroimaging techniques play a critical role in assessing the effectiveness of therapeutic interventions, such as pharmacological treatments or deep brain stimulation (DBS). For instance, MRI and PET scans are employed to evaluate the effects of disease-modifying treatments in AD and to assess changes in brain metabolism in response to treatments in PD.

Biomarker Development: Neuroimaging is integral in identifying biomarkers that can predict therapeutic outcomes. The use of amyloid imaging to monitor the effects of anti-amyloid therapies in AD is a prime example.

4. Future directions in neuroimaging

The field of neuroimaging is continuously evolving, and several emerging technologies hold promise for enhancing the diagnosis and treatment of neurodegenerative diseases.

4.1 Multimodal imaging

The integration of multiple neuroimaging modalities, such as combining PET and MRI, holds significant potential for more comprehensive assessments of neurodegenerative diseases. Multimodal imaging can provide both structural and functional information, offering a more detailed view of disease mechanisms and progression.

4.2 Neuroimaging biomarkers in clinical trials

The use of neuroimaging biomarkers in clinical trials is rapidly expanding. These biomarkers are being utilized to monitor disease progression and therapeutic response, aiding in the development of new drugs. Furthermore, neuroimaging is increasingly important in precision medicine by identifying patient subgroups that are most likely to benefit from specific treatments [79].

4.3 Artificial intelligence (AI) and machine learning in neuroimaging

AI and machine learning algorithms are beginning to revolutionize the field of neuroimaging. These technologies are being used to automate the analysis of neuroimaging data, improve diagnostic accuracy, and predict disease progression. For example, deep learning algorithms can be trained to recognize patterns in MRI scans that predict the onset of neurodegenerative diseases even before clinical symptoms appear. Integrating artificial intelligence (AI) in neuroimaging transforms data analysis, enabling automated detection and quantification of pathological changes. Machine learning algorithms improve diagnostic accuracy and streamline workflow efficiency [81].

4.4 Functional neuroimaging and disease mechanisms

Advances in functional neuroimaging, such as resting-state fMRI and task-based fMRI, offer new insights into the dynamic changes in brain networks associated with neurodegenerative diseases. Understanding how these networks are altered will provide critical information for developing targeted treatments.

4.5 Advanced imaging modalities

Emerging technologies, such as ultrahigh-field MRI and photon-counting CT, offer superior resolution and contrast, unveiling previously inaccessible details of brain pathology. These advancements hold promise for enhancing diagnostic and therapeutic precision [82].

4.6 Therapeutic neuroimaging

Real-time neuroimaging during interventional procedures, such as deep brain stimulation (DBS) or focused ultrasound, enables precise targeting and monitoring of therapeutic interventions. These advancements are pivotal in optimizing outcomes and minimizing risks [81].

5. Conclusion

Interventional neuroimaging is rapidly evolving, with transformative potential in diagnosing and treating neurodegenerative diseases. Emerging technologies such as advanced MRI techniques, real-time image-guided interventions, and AI-driven data analysis enhance precision, improve patient outcomes, and enable minimally invasive procedures. The future of interventional neuroimaging lies in its ability to integrate with personalized medicine, optimize therapeutic strategies, and support early detection of neurological disorders. Continued interdisciplinary collaboration and technological innovation will be key drivers in advancing clinical applications, ultimately reshaping patient care in neuroscience.

Author details

Naheed Akhter, Sadia Sana*, Yasmin Mushtaq, Mamoona Tariq and Maryam Afzaal
College of Allied Health Professionals, Directorate of Medical Sciences, Govt. College University, Faisalabad, Pakistan

*Address all correspondence to: sadiasana203@gmail.com

References

[1] Erkkinen MG, Kim M-O, Geschwind MD. Clinical neurology and epidemiology of the major neurodegenerative diseases. Cold Spring Harbor Perspectives in Biology. 2018;**10**(4):a033118

[2] Dugger BN, Dickson DW. Pathology of neurodegenerative diseases. Cold Spring Harbor Perspectives in Biology. 2017;**9**(7):a028035

[3] Liu H et al. Mendelian randomization highlights significant difference and genetic heterogeneity in clinically diagnosed Alzheimer's disease GWAS and self-report proxy phenotype GWAX. Alzheimer's Research & Therapy. 2022;**14**(1):17

[4] Onohuean H et al. Epidemiology of neurodegenerative diseases in the east African region: A meta-analysis. Frontiers in Neurology. 2022;**13**:1024004

[5] Bruzova M et al. Autopsy-diagnosed neurodegenerative dementia cases support the use of cerebrospinal fluid protein biomarkers in the diagnostic work-up. Scientific Reports. 2021;**11**(1):10837

[6] Pansarasa O et al. Biomarkers in human peripheral blood mononuclear cells: The state of the art in amyotrophic lateral sclerosis. International Journal of Molecular Sciences. 2022;**23**(5):2580

[7] Singla RK et al. Natural kinase inhibitors for the treatment and management of endometrial/uterine cancer: Preclinical to clinical studies. Frontiers in Pharmacology. 2022;**13**:801733

[8] Chopra H et al. Chemopreventive potential of dietary nanonutraceuticals for prostate cancer: An extensive review. Frontiers in Oncology. 2022;**12**:925379

[9] Karim N et al. Natural products as an emerging therapeutic alternative in the treatment of neurological disorders. Evidence-based Complementary and Alternative Medicine. 2018;**2018**:1-2

[10] Singla RK et al. Natural products for the management of castration-resistant prostate cancer: Special focus on nanoparticles based studies. Frontiers in Cell and Developmental Biology. 2021;**9**:745177

[11] Patel SS, Udayabanu M. Effect of natural products on diabetes associated neurological disorders. Reviews in the Neurosciences. 2017;**28**(3):271-293

[12] Rahman MH et al. Therapeutic potential of natural products in treating neurodegenerative disorders and their future prospects and challenges. Molecules. 2021;**26**(17):5327

[13] Singh A et al. Oxidative stress: A key modulator in neurodegenerative diseases. Molecules. 2019;**24**(8):1583

[14] Radi R. Oxygen radicals, nitric oxide, and peroxynitrite: Redox pathways in molecular medicine. Proceedings of the National Academy of Sciences. 2018;**115**(23):5839-5848

[15] de Almeida AJPO et al. ROS: Basic concepts, sources, cellular signaling, and its implications in aging pathways. Oxidative Medicine and Cellular Longevity. 2022;**2022**(1):1225578

[16] Tirichen H et al. Mitochondrial reactive oxygen species and their contribution in chronic kidney disease progression through oxidative stress. Frontiers in Physiology. 2021;**12**:627837

[17] Teleanu DM et al. An overview of oxidative stress, neuroinflammation, and neurodegenerative diseases. International Journal of Molecular Sciences. 2022;**23**(11):5938

[18] Gitler AD, Dhillon P, Shorter J. Neurodegenerative disease: Models, mechanisms, and a new hope. Disease Models & Mechanisms. 2017;**10**(5):499-502

[19] Federico A et al. Mitochondria, oxidative stress and neurodegeneration. Journal of the Neurological Sciences. 2012;**322**(1-2):254-262

[20] Martin LJ. Biology of mitochondria in neurodegenerative diseases. Progress in Molecular Biology and Translational Science. 2012;**107**:355-415

[21] Kühlbrandt W. Structure and function of mitochondrial membrane protein complexes. BMC Biology. 2015;**13**:1-11

[22] Westermann B. Bioenergetic role of mitochondrial fusion and fission. Biochimica et Biophysica Acta (BBA)-Bioenergetics. 2012;**1817**(10):1833-1838

[23] Onyango IG, Dennis J, Khan SM. Mitochondrial dysfunction in Alzheimer's disease and the rationale for bioenergetics based therapies. Aging and Disease. 2016;7(2):201

[24] Masters CL et al. Alzheimer's disease. Nature Reviews Disease Primers. 2015;**1**(1):1-18

[25] Scheltens P et al. Alzheimer's disease. The Lancet. 2016;**388**(10043):505-517

[26] Poewe W et al. Parkinson's disease. Nature Reviews Disease Primers. 2017;**3**(1):1-21

[27] Soto C. Protein misfolding and disease; protein refolding and therapy. FEBS Letters. 2001;**498**(2-3):204-207

[28] Kelly JW. Alternative conformations of amyloidogenic proteins govern their behavior. Current Opinion in Structural Biology. 1996;**6**(1):11-17

[29] Stoessl AJ. Neuroimaging in the early diagnosis of neurodegenerative disease. Translational Neurodegeneration. 2012;**1**:1-6

[30] Blennow K, Zetterberg H, Fagan AM. Fluid biomarkers in Alzheimer disease. Cold Spring Harbor Perspectives in Medicine. 2012;**2**(9):a006221

[31] Pais MV, Forlenza OV, Diniz BS. Plasma biomarkers of Alzheimer's disease: A review of available assays, recent developments, and implications for clinical practice. Journal of Alzheimer's Disease Reports. 2023;7(1):355-380

[32] Hong-Qi Y, Zhi-Kun S, Sheng-Di C. Current advances in the treatment of Alzheimer's disease: Focused on considerations targeting Aβ and tau. Translational Neurodegeneration. 2012;**1**:1-12

[33] Roberson ED, Mucke L. 100 years and counting: Prospects for defeating Alzheimer's disease. Science. 2006;**314**(5800):781-784

[34] Sharma A, Bemis M, Desilets AR. Role of medium chain triglycerides (Axona®) in the treatment of mild to moderate Alzheimer's disease. American Journal of Alzheimer's Disease & Other Dementias®. 2014;**29**(5):409-414

[35] Jankovic J. Levodopa strengths and weaknesses. Neurology. 2002;**58**(suppl_1):S19-S32

[36] Korczyn A et al. A 3-year randomized trial of ropinirole and bromocriptine in early Parkinson's disease. Neurology. 1999;**53**(2):364-364

[37] Yao LH et al. Flavonoids in food and their health benefits. Plant Foods for Human Nutrition. 2004;**59**:113-122

[38] Sandoval-Acuña C, Ferreira J, Speisky H. Polyphenols and mitochondria: An update on their increasingly emerging ROS-scavenging independent actions. Archives of Biochemistry and Biophysics. 2014;**559**:75-90

[39] Smolensky D et al. High-polyphenol sorghum bran extract inhibits cancer cell growth through ROS induction, cell cycle arrest, and apoptosis. Journal of Medicinal Food. 2018;**21**(10):990-998

[40] Kinarivala N et al. Discovery of aromatic carbamates that confer neuroprotective activity by enhancing autophagy and inducing the anti-apoptotic protein B-cell lymphoma 2 (Bcl-2). Journal of Medicinal Chemistry. 2017;**60**(23):9739-9756

[41] Di Meo F et al. New therapeutic drugs from bioactive natural molecules: The role of gut microbiota metabolism in neurodegenerative diseases. Current Drug Metabolism. 2018;**19**(6):478-489

[42] Redza-Dutordoir M, Averill-Bates DA. Activation of apoptosis signalling pathways by reactive oxygen species. Biochimica et Biophysica Acta (BBA)-Molecular Cell Research. 2016;**1863**(12):2977-2992

[43] Vacínová G et al. Regulated upon activation, normal T cell expressed and secreted (RANTES) levels in the peripheral blood of patients with Alzheimer's disease. Neural Regeneration Research. 2021;**16**(4):796-800

[44] Qin S, Hou DX. Multiple regulations of Keap1/Nrf2 system by dietary phytochemicals. Molecular Nutrition & Food Research. 2016;**60**(8):1731-1755

[45] Gheldof N, Engeseth NJ. Antioxidant capacity of honeys from various floral sources based on the determination of oxygen radical absorbance capacity and inhibition of in vitro lipoprotein oxidation in human serum samples. Journal of Agricultural and Food Chemistry. 2002;**50**(10):3050-3055

[46] Tungmunnithum D et al. Flavonoids and other phenolic compounds from medicinal plants for pharmaceutical and medical aspects: An overview. Medicine. 2018;**5**(3):93

[47] Ak T, Gülçin I. Antioxidant and radical scavenging properties of curcumin. Chemico-Biological Interactions. 2008;**174**(1):27-37

[48] Foley TD. Reductive reprogramming: A not-so-radical hypothesis of neurodegeneration linking redox perturbations to neuroinflammation and excitotoxicity. Cellular and Molecular Neurobiology. 2019;**39**(5):577-590

[49] Cui K et al. Role of oxidative stress in neurodegeneration: Recent developments in assay methods for oxidative stress and nutraceutical antioxidants. Progress in Neuro-Psychopharmacology and Biological Psychiatry. 2004;**28**(5):771-799

[50] Mattson MP, Magnus T. Ageing and neuronal vulnerability. Nature Reviews Neuroscience. 2006;**7**(4):278-294

[51] Kim SJ et al. Curcumin stimulates proliferation of embryonic neural progenitor cells and neurogenesis in the adult hippocampus. Journal of Biological Chemistry. 2008;**283**(21):14497-14505

[52] Yuan H et al. The protective effects of resveratrol on Schwann cells with toxicity induced by ethanol in vitro. Neurochemistry International. 2013;**63**(3):146-153

[53] Di Pardo A et al. Impairment of blood-brain barrier is an early event in R6/2 mouse model of Huntington disease. Scientific Reports. 2017;**7**(1):41316

[54] Andrieu S et al. Prevention of sporadic Alzheimer's disease: Lessons learned from clinical trials and future directions. The Lancet Neurology. 2015;**14**(9):926-944

[55] Querfurth HW, LaFerla FM. Mechanisms of disease. The New England Journal of Medicine. 2010;**362**(4):329-344

[56] Rezai-Zadeh K et al. Green tea epigallocatechin-3-gallate (EGCG) reduces β-amyloid mediated cognitive impairment and modulates tau pathology in Alzheimer transgenic mice. Brain Research. 2008;**1214**:177-187

[57] Zhang X et al. Quercetin stabilizes apolipoprotein E and reduces brain Aβ levels in amyloid model mice. Neuropharmacology. 2016;**108**:179-192

[58] Alexander GE. Biology of Parkinson's disease: Pathogenesis and pathophysiology of a multisystem neurodegenerative disorder. Dialogues in Clinical Neuroscience. 2004;**6**(3):259-280

[59] Miller RL, Sun GY, Sun AY. Cytotoxicity of paraquat in microglial cells: Involvement of PKCδ-and ERK1/2-dependent NADPH oxidase. Brain Research. 2007;**1167**:129-139

[60] Ramkumar M et al. Demethoxycurcumin ameliorates rotenone-induced toxicity in rats. Frontiers in Bioscience-Elite. 2019;**11**(1):1-11

[61] Wang Y-L et al. Protective effect of curcumin against oxidative stress-induced injury in rats with Parkinson's disease through the Wnt/β-catenin signaling pathway. Cellular Physiology and Biochemistry. 2017;**43**(6):2226-2241

[62] Yu S et al. Curcumin exerts anti-inflammatory and antioxidative properties in 1-methyl-4-phenylpyridinium ion (MPP+)-stimulated mesencephalic astrocytes by interference with TLR4 and downstream signaling pathway. Cell Stress and Chaperones. 2016;**21**(4):697-705

[63] Potdar S et al. Protective effects of the resveratrol analog piceid in dopaminergic SH-SY5Y cells. Archives of Toxicology. 2018;**92**:669-677

[64] Walker FO. Huntington's disease. The Lancet. 2007;**369**(9557):218-228

[65] Sciacca S et al. Early enteric neuron dysfunction in mouse and human Huntington disease. Parkinsonism & Related Disorders. 2017;**34**:73-74

[66] Chakraborty J et al. Quercetin improves behavioral deficiencies, restores astrocytes and microglia, and reduces serotonin metabolism in 3-nitropropionic acid-induced rat model of Huntington's disease. CNS Neuroscience & Therapeutics. 2014;**20**(1):10-19

[67] Anastacio JR et al. Resveratrol treatment has neuroprotective effects and prevents cognitive impairment after chronic cerebral hypoperfusion. Neurological Research. 2014;**36**(7):627-633

[68] Shen D et al. Effect of melatonin and resveratrol against memory impairment and hippocampal damage in a rat model of vascular dementia. Neuroimmunomodulation. 2017;**23**(5-6):318-331

[69] Tota S et al. Protective effect of quercetin against intracerebral

streptozotocin induced reduction in cerebral blood flow and impairment of memory in mice. Behavioural Brain Research. 2010;**209**(1):73-79

[70] Murumulla L, Challa S. Role of apoptosis in neurodegeneration: Therapeutic targets and strategies. In: Apoptosis and Human Health: Understanding Mechanistic and Therapeutic Potential. Cham, Switzerland: Springer; 2024. pp. 231-249

[71] Wang H et al. Neuroimaging techniques, gene therapy, and gut microbiota: Frontier advances and integrated applications in Alzheimer's disease research. Frontiers in Aging Neuroscience. 2024;**16**:1485657

[72] Kitson SL. Modern Medical Imaging and Radiation Therapy. Cyber Security| Big Data| AI. Open Med Science. 2024

[73] Mannheim JG et al. PET/MRI hybrid systems. In: Seminars in Nuclear Medicine. Elsevier; 2018

[74] Alanazi MMF, Alhebs MA. Advancements in hybrid imaging techniques: Enhancing diagnostic accuracy with PET/MRI and PET/CT. International Journal of Health Sciences. 1800;**8**(S1):1800-1811

[75] Garibotto V et al. Molecular neuroimaging with PET/MRI. Clinical and Translational Imaging. 2013;**1**:53-63

[76] Zuo C et al. Molecular imaging for neurological diseases. In: Transpathology. Elsevier; 2024. pp. 247-258

[77] Catana C et al. MRI-assisted PET motion correction for neurologic studies in an integrated MR-PET scanner. Journal of Nuclear Medicine. 2011;**52**(1):154-161

[78] Lee J et al. Current trends and applications of PET/MRI hybrid imaging in neurodegenerative diseases and Normal aging. Diagnostics. 2024;**14**(6):585

[79] Aiello M et al. Neuroinflammation in neurodegenerative diseases: Current multi-modal imaging studies and future opportunities for hybrid PET/MRI. Neuroscience. 2019;**403**:125-135

[80] Ibrahim AA, Alghamdi ASM. The Role of Hybrid Imaging Techniques in Improving the Accuracy of Tumor Diagnosis

[81] Weida MJ, Yee B. Quantum cascade laser-based replacement for FTIR microscopy. In: Imaging, Manipulation, and Analysis of Biomolecules, Cells, and Tissues IX. SPIE; 2011

[82] Saylor MJ. The Mobile Wave: How Mobile Intelligence Will Change Everything. Hachette+ ORM; 2013

Chapter 6

Neuronavigation: Neuroimaging Applied to Neuromodulation and Neurosurgery

Chiara Di Fazio and Sara Palermo

Abstract

Neuronavigation has revolutionised neurosurgery by enabling precise targeting of brain structures through the integration of real-time surgical navigation and advanced neuroimaging (CT, magnetic resonance imaging (MRI), fMRI). Recent advances in infrared and electromagnetic technology have improved preoperative assessment, surgical planning and intraoperative guidance for procedures such as biopsies, tumour resections and deep brain stimulation (DBS). This chapter focuses on structural and functional neuroimaging modalities and their applications in surgical planning and execution. It also examines how neuronavigation contributes to neuromodulation techniques (DBS, transcranial magnetic stimulation (TMS)), tumour resection and epilepsy surgery. Emerging technologies such as resting-state fMRI and portable imaging systems for the operating theatre (POSITs) are discussed. The chapter concludes with an outlook on future developments, including the integration of artificial intelligence, machine learning and augmented/virtual reality to further improve accuracy and efficiency in neurosurgical practice. The continued integration of neuroimaging remains critical to optimising neurosurgical outcomes.

Keywords: neuronavigation, neuroimaging, neurosurgery, neuromodulation, deep brain stimulation, fMRI, tumour resection, epilepsy surgery

1. Introduction

The advent of neuronavigation has transformed neurosurgery, ushering in an era of unprecedented precision in navigating the intricate structures of the brain [1]. By integrating real-time surgical navigation with advanced neuroimaging technologies such as computed tomography (CT), magnetic resonance imaging (MRI) and functional MRI (fMRI), neuronavigation significantly minimises the risks associated with surgical procedures and improves patient outcomes [2, 3].

Recent advances in infrared and electromagnetic technology have further expanded the possibilities of neuronavigation [4, 5]. Compact, multifunctional electromagnetic navigation systems now enhance preoperative assessment, surgical planning, and intraoperative guidance. These innovations optimise procedures such as biopsies, tumour excision, and radiofrequency ablation, improving both precision and efficiency [6].

In the past, limited access to neuroimaging data during surgery posed a challenge and occasionally hindered important intraoperative decisions. In response, frameless stereotactic neurosurgery has evolved towards value-based image registration, overcoming the limitations of traditional feature detection algorithms [2, 3, 6, 7]. Innovative software platforms now enable better classification during surgical procedures and offer improved predictions of ablation zones and tissue necrosis assessments. As a result, neuronavigation supports the customisation of surgical procedures to the specific anatomical and pathological characteristics of each patient [3, 8].

In addition to tumour resection, neuronavigation plays a crucial role in a number of neurosurgical procedures, including deep brain stimulation (DBS) [1, 5, 9]. Modern methods include specialised tools that divide the planning phase into systematic steps and optimise access routes for the placement of electrodes. In many operating theatres today, advanced navigation systems are used for preoperative modelling and precise electrode placement, with cryogenically cooled electrodes providing even greater precision [1–9].

Given its growing number of applications, the continued prioritisation of neuroimaging in neuronavigation is essential. This chapter aims to provide a comprehensive overview of the principles, advances and future directions of neuronavigation in modern neurosurgery, with a particular focus on its application in neuromodulation and general neurosurgery.

1.1 Overview of neuronavigation

Neuronavigation represents a transformative technology in neurosurgery, enabling unprecedented accuracy through the integration of imaging techniques such as CT, MRI, and fMRI [2]. These modalities enable targeted interventions for a range of neurological and psychiatric disorders, particularly in neuromodulation applications [3, 5].

The global neurosurgical community increasingly relies on neuronavigation for intraoperative guidance, enhancing surgical precision and decision-making confidence [1, 3, 5, 8]. Traditional CT imaging has evolved to support real-time preoperative strategies, while MRI and resting-state fMRI provide complementary structural and functional insights, further augmenting neuronavigation's efficacy [10]. Modern MRI techniques offer multi-planar views with unparalleled clarity, empowering surgeons with comprehensive anatomical visualisation [11–16].

Despite its advancements, literature on the technological frameworks underpinning neuronavigation—such as CT control room configurations—remains limited. Expanding knowledge of patient-specific anatomy and neurovascular landmarks is critical to improving surgical accuracy and minimising iatrogenic risks [2, 7, 17].

A critical component of neuronavigation is the computer workstation, which processes multimodal imaging data to generate real-time, dynamic representations of brain structures. This integration enables surgeons to navigate anatomical regions with unprecedented clarity. Additionally, portable operating room imaging systems (POSITs) enhance intraoperative imaging accessibility, incorporating cost functions and dose analysis models to autonomously compute hazard zones, target positions, and trajectory paths [18–20]. Innovations such as super-compact laser actuation systems further refine stereotactic neuronavigation, compensating for slight head deviations and enhancing surgical precision [21, 22]. Laser guidance technologies, coupled with photon detectors tracking head position in three-dimensional space, ensure real-time synchronisation of anatomical representations, advancing surgical motility and accuracy [23]. These developments herald a new era in neurosurgery, characterised by unparalleled precision and improved patient outcomes.

1.1.1 Hardware and software components

A typical neuronavigation system consists of [24–26]:

- *Workstation:* the heart of the system, a powerful computing unit that processes neuroimaging data and displays navigation information in real time. Modern workstations are equipped with high-performance processors, large RAM capacity and special graphics cards to process large amounts of image data and 3D rendering. The most common operating systems are Windows or Linux with intuitive and customisable user interfaces. Specialised software enables preoperative planning, patient registration and intraoperative navigation.

- *Tracking system*: This component tracks the position of the surgical instruments and the patient in space. The most common systems include.

    - *Infrared (IR):* Infrared cameras detect the position of reflective (passive) or emitting (active) markers attached to the instruments and patient. IR systems offer high precision and fast tracking but are susceptible to visual obstructions.

    - *Electromagnetic (EM):* A magnetic field generated by a transmitter is used to track the position of sensors attached to the instruments. EM systems are less affected by visual obstructions compared to IR systems and allow a wider tracking range but can be affected by metallic interference.

- *User interface:* A high-resolution monitor displays neuroimaging (MRI, CT, PET), the position of the surgical instruments superimposed on the images and other relevant information (e.g. distances to the target and approach angle). Modern user interfaces are interactive and allow the surgeon to manipulate images, plan trajectories and visualise 3D information.

- *Surgical instruments:* Instruments specifically designed to be tracked by the navigation system. These may include probes, suction devices, electrodes for deep brain stimulation (DBS) and other procedure-specific instruments.

- *Surgical planning software:* Specialised software enables preoperative planning, patient registration and intraoperative navigation. Advanced features include multimodal image fusion, anatomical structure segmentation, surgical simulation and 3D visualisation. Examples of surgical planning software include:

    - *Brainlab Elements:* A comprehensive suite of software modules for various neurosurgical applications, including tumour surgery planning, DBS planning and spine surgery planning. It integrates with Brainlab's navigation systems and offers features such as automatic trajectory planning, 3D visualisation and surgical simulation.

    - *Medtronic StealthStation:* A surgical navigation system that includes preoperative planning software and intraoperative tracking. The StealthStation software enables multimodal image fusion, anatomical segmentation and trajectory planning. The tracking system uses infrared cameras to precisely localise surgical instruments.

- o *Other software:* Other surgical planning platforms include Surgical Theatre SNAP, Siemens syngo.via and Philips IntelliSpace Portal.

These components work together to increase surgical precision, improve patient outcomes and support complex neurosurgical procedures.

2. Neuroimaging techniques

Neuroimaging has revolutionised modern neurosurgery and enables more precise interventions through better visualisation of brain structures and functions. Advanced imaging techniques have enabled surgical procedures previously thought impossible and improved both inpatient and outpatient outcomes [2, 3].

Structural imaging modalities such as MRI and 4D flow MRI provide critical insights into the architecture of the brain and cerebral blood supply and serve as a benchmark for pathology definitions and patient safety [11–14, 27, 28]. Functional imaging techniques such as fMRI and PET help to understand brain activity and inform surgical decisions. [10, 29–31]

The integration of these imaging modalities enables neurosurgeons to develop comprehensive preoperative strategies that ensure safer and more effective surgical interventions. In addition, real-time imaging enhancements, such as 3D visualisations and film loops, provide dynamic representations of blood flow and neural networks that further improve surgical precision.

2.1 Structural imaging

Accurate neurosurgical planning requires detailed anatomical maps tailored to each patient's unique brain structure. In the past, structural imaging modalities provided relatively low-resolution images. However, recent advances in imaging technology have significantly improved resolution and expanded their clinical applications [7, 32].

Modern MRI and CT techniques utilise a variety of imaging parameters, including T1/T2 relaxation times, diffusion coefficients and angiogenesis markers, to produce a highly detailed representation of brain anatomy. While MRI is known for its superior contrast resolution [33], CT remains indispensable due to its accessibility and fast acquisition times, especially in emergency situations where timely intervention is critical.

The integration of high-resolution imaging data into neuronavigation systems has significantly improved diagnostic accuracy and surgical precision. Nevertheless, it remains a challenge to achieve sub-millimetre accuracy in complex procedures. Overcoming these limitations requires constant innovation in imaging technology and the expertise of experienced radiologists to effectively interpret high-resolution data sets [1].

2.2 Functional imaging

Functional imaging techniques have become indispensable in modern neurosurgery. They provide insights into brain activity and facilitate the identification of critical functional areas prior to surgical interventions [35]. Among the most widely used modalities are fMRI and PET, both of which provide valuable information about brain function and metabolic processes.

fMRI utilises blood oxygenation level-dependent contrast (BOLD) to measure changes in cerebral blood flow associated with neuronal activity. This non-invasive technique allows neurosurgeons to image functional areas of the brain, such as language and motor regions, improving preoperative planning and minimising the risk of postoperative deficits [7, 10, 33–34]. In addition, resting-state fMRI has proven to be a powerful tool for assessing functional connectivity within brain networks, providing further information on surgical strategies.

Resting-state fMRI (rs-fMRI) has proven to be a valuable tool for identifying intrinsic connectivity networks in the brain and provides unique insights into functional organisation [36]. In contrast to task-based fMRI, rs-fMRI measures brain activity in the resting state, revealing patterns of correlated activity between different brain regions. This is particularly beneficial in identifying eloquent areas and assessing the impact of lesions on brain networks, which can aid in surgical planning and risk assessment [37–38].

PET imaging, on the other hand, provides insights into metabolic activity through the detection of radiolabelled tracers that bind to specific biological targets. This method is particularly useful in identifying tumour characteristics and distinguishing between different tumour types, as well as in assessing brain metabolism in neurodegenerative diseases [39]. In combination with structural imaging techniques, PET can provide a comprehensive understanding of both the anatomical and functional aspects of brain pathology [40].

The integration of functional imaging into neuronavigation systems has significantly improved surgical precision by enabling real-time visualisation of critical functional areas during surgery. However, standardisation of protocols and interpretation of complex data sets remain a challenge. Continued advances in imaging technologies and analysis methods will be critical to optimising the benefits of functional imaging in neurosurgery.

3. Applications in neuromodulation

Neuromodulation techniques such as deep brain stimulation (DBS) and transcranial magnetic stimulation (TMS) have proven to be promising approaches for the treatment of a range of neurological and psychiatric disorders. Neuronavigation plays a crucial role in guiding and improving the precision of these interventions, thereby improving therapeutic outcomes.

In DBS, electrodes are implanted in specific regions of the brain to modulate neural circuits [41, 42]. Neuronavigation is essential for the precise placement of the electrodes. It ensures that the targeted brain structures are reached precisely while minimising the risk of damage to the surrounding tissue [43, 44]. Preoperative planning with MRI and CT imaging combined with intraoperative guidance by neuronavigation systems allows neurosurgeons to navigate the complex anatomy of the brain and place the electrodes with sub-millimetre accuracy.

Transcranial magnetic stimulation is a non-invasive neuromodulation technique in which magnetic pulses are used to stimulate or inhibit neuronal activity in specific regions of the brain [45]. Neuronavigation is used to direct the TMS coil to the desired cortical area, which enables precise and reproducible stimulation [46]. TMS controlled by neuronavigation has proven promising in the treatment of depression, obsessive-compulsive disorder and chronic pain, among others.

The integration of neuronavigation into neuromodulation techniques has revolutionised the treatment of neurological and psychiatric disorders, providing physicians with more precise and effective tools. Recent studies have highlighted the role of neuroplasticity in neuromodulatory interventions, highlighting how TMS and DBS can induce long-term synaptic changes in motor and cognitive networks [47–49].

For example, TMS-induced modulation of the prefrontal cortex has been associated with improved executive function and emotion regulation in both clinical and ageing populations, underscoring the importance of individualising stimulation protocols based on patient-specific functional connectivity profiles networks [47–49]. However, the optimisation of stimulation parameters and the personalisation of treatment strategies remains a challenge [46]. Further research and technological advances are needed to further improve the efficacy and safety of neuromodulation interventions (**Figure 1**).

3.1 Deep brain stimulation

DBS represents an advanced neuromodulation method that successfully addresses a variety of neurological conditions resistant to medication, including Parkinson's disease, epilepsy, OCD, chronic pain, and Tourette's syndrome. As an illustration of this, one can analyse what DBS has accomplished, which involves inserting and positioning fine wires and electrodes in precisely defined areas of the brain and subsequent delivery of controlled electrical impulses with pinpoint accuracy [41, 42].

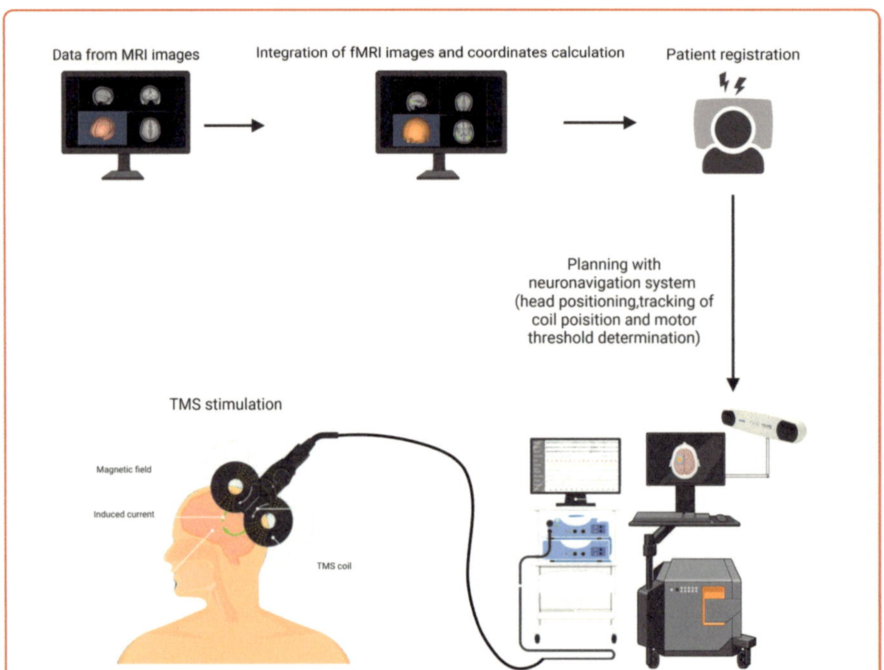

Figure 1.
Neuronavigation platform used in a transcranial magnetic stimulation (TMS) setting. The figure shows a complete neuronavigation setup for the precise localization of cortical targets during non-invasive neuromodulation treatments. This technology enables individualized stimulation based on the patient's anatomical features.

This process enables the adjustment of faulty electrical activity in the brain, resulting in symptomatic improvement.

By employing high-resolution neuroimaging techniques (like MRI or CT scans), this technology creates high-resolution anatomical maps of brain areas to allow for accurate localisation of targets in the brain [9, 43, 44]. Mapping in the preoperative phase makes it possible for neurosurgeons to select optimal electrode insertion sites on movement areas of the brain, particularly in the subthalamic region (STN), which is crucial for the regulation of motor functions [9, 50, 51].

The accuracy offered by neuronavigation enhances the chance of achieving clinical targets while lowering the risk of procedural complications by using real-time imaging. By preventing intraoperative complications such as hematomas and air intrusions, this capability plays a crucial role in enhancing patient safety [43, 44].

Notwithstanding the accomplishments of DBS, individual patient variability means that stimulation parameters often require modification postoperatively. Neuronavigation helps doctors to carefully track and adjust these parameters in real time according to the patient's changing responses, leading to personalised treatment and reduced toxicity. Moreover, advances in the standardisation of these modifications will ultimately provide a better opportunity for personalised care and increase the longevity and effectiveness of DBS.

3.2 Transcranial magnetic stimulation

Neuronavigation improves the efficacy and accuracy of transcranial magnetic stimulation (TMS), a non-invasive neuromodulation technique that uses magnetic fields to stimulate specific regions of the brain [46, 52]. TMS was developed in the 1990s and has been shown to be highly beneficial for mental health and various neurological disorders [45, 46]. Unlike invasive surgical procedures such as DBS, where electrodes are implanted to deliver electrical current, TMS therapy is performed on an outpatient basis, making it a less invasive alternative [45, 46]. Neuronavigation is critical to ensure that the TMS pulses are delivered precisely to the desired cortical target.

TMS exerts its therapeutic effect by repeatedly sending magnetic pulses to the scalp, thereby modulating electrical activity in the underlying brain regions. When directed to the motor cortex (precentral gyrus), it can elicit perceptible motor responses, demonstrating its potential for studying brain function. Neuronavigation improves the consistency and reliability of this targeting [53]. The integration of neuronavigation with repetitive TMS (rTMS) has significantly enhanced targeting accuracy, leading to improved treatment outcomes in neuropsychiatric disorders networks [47–49]. This is particularly evident in disorders such as major depression, where precise dorsolateral prefrontal cortex stimulation has shown higher response rates compared to non-navigated approaches. Additionally, the use of functional neuroimaging to personalise coil positioning has further refined stimulation strategies, optimising therapeutic efficacy while minimising variability.

Single-pulse TMS is mainly used in research, while rTMS is favoured in therapy to achieve long-lasting changes in brain activity with longer series of pulses. Low-frequency rTMS (1 Hz) suppresses activity, while high-frequency rTMS ($\geq$ 5 Hz) has an excitatory effect [54]. Neuronavigation improves the precision of target localisation in rTMS, which translates into better treatment outcomes for various conditions. In medical areas where accuracy is critical — such as mood disorders, chronic pain, cognitive rehabilitation and stroke recovery — stimulating the relevant areas of the brain with neuronavigation can lead to more predictable outcomes [52, 54].

The FDA has approved rTMS for treatment-resistant major depressive disorder and is evaluating its use for obsessive-compulsive disorder [55–56]. Current studies are also investigating the efficacy of rTMS for neuropathic pain and stroke recovery. Intermittent theta burst stimulation (iTBS), a newer therapy, has received FDA approval. It is just as effective as rTMS but requires shorter session durations. Neuronavigation plays a crucial role in the accurate delivery of iTBS to the target region. While rTMS has shown promising potential, the heterogeneity of the results obtained in the different studies emphasises the need for refined treatment protocols, better identification of patients who could benefit from treatment and more convincing evidence of the efficacy of the therapy in different conditions. Neuronavigation helps to reduce this variability by improving targeting accuracy.

TMS offers a powerful non-invasive option for modulating brain function and serves as an alternative for patients who cannot undergo more invasive procedures such as DBS, especially with the help of neuronavigation technology.

3.3 MRI guided focussed ultrasound

Magnetic resonance-guided focussed ultrasound (MRgFUS) has become a rapidly advancing non-invasive method in neurosurgery that enables non-invasive thermal ablation of deep brain areas [56]. This technique, which enables non-invasive thermal ablation of deep brain areas, combines the accuracy of focussed ultrasound energy with the accuracy of real-time MRI imaging. MRgFUS is considered an acceptable alternative to conventional surgery as it is less invasive and allows localised treatment without surgical incisions. Similar to frameless stereotaxy in traditional neurosurgery, MRgFUS relies on accurate registration of the patient's anatomy in a preoperative image dataset [56].

By focussing ultrasound waves on specific regions of the brain, MRgFUS offers a promising new treatment method. MRI enables precise treatment planning and real-time monitoring, analogous to intraoperative imaging updates in open neuronavigation procedures. This real-time monitoring allows for better control of the treatment process and immediate adjustments based on tissue response. This is a key aspect of neuronavigation – adjusting the surgical strategy based on intraoperative feedback.

In addition, MR thermography, often in conjunction with ceramic cooling systems with disposable water buffers, allows for better thermal management during the procedure, reducing the likelihood of overheating and the resulting thermal effects.

Focussed ultrasound has been used to effectively ablate thalamic regions responsible for controlling tremors in patients with Parkinson's disease and Essential Tremor (ET) [57]. The FDA has approved MRgFUS for essential tremor (ET) to help patients for whom medical therapy has failed or who wish to avoid a more invasive surgical procedure.

Each patient is positioned in an MRI suite and wears a special helmet that directs the ultrasound beams to the target regions in the brain. This helmet and the MRI guidance system act as a form of non-invasive neuronavigation. In clinical practice, MRgFUS is increasingly being used for a growing range of neurological conditions, including the treatment of tremors in Parkinson's disease. The amount of tissue ablated is critical to the success of the procedure, and advanced imaging allows physicians to visualise the ablation in real time, providing important data on the effectiveness of the treatment. This real-time feedback loop is a hallmark of effective neuronavigation.

The thalamus is often the target of interventions to relieve symptoms, emphasising the need for immediate assessment of the impact of MRgFUS on tremor therapy [57].

Although the procedure is minimally invasive, patient selection is critical to its efficacy. Technical and non-technical factors such as facial twitching, head movements and sonication techniques can negatively impact treatment outcomes [57]. Advanced motion correction algorithms, like those used in neuronavigation, are being developed to mitigate the effects of these factors.

These models, combined with precise targeting and real-time feedback, are an example of the future of personalised, image-guided interventions that align with the core principles of neuronavigation.

4. Applications in neurosurgery

Neuronavigation has transformed neurosurgical interventions by enabling real-time visualisation of brain structures during procedures. This technology is particularly valuable in tumour resection, epilepsy surgery, and functional neurosurgery (**Figure 2**).

4.1 Tumour resection

Neuronavigation is changing tumour resection by moving from vague surgical approaches to precisely defined parameters that increase surgical readiness. Neurosurgeons equipped with neuronavigation can precisely define resection margins, maximising safe tumour removal while protecting surrounding

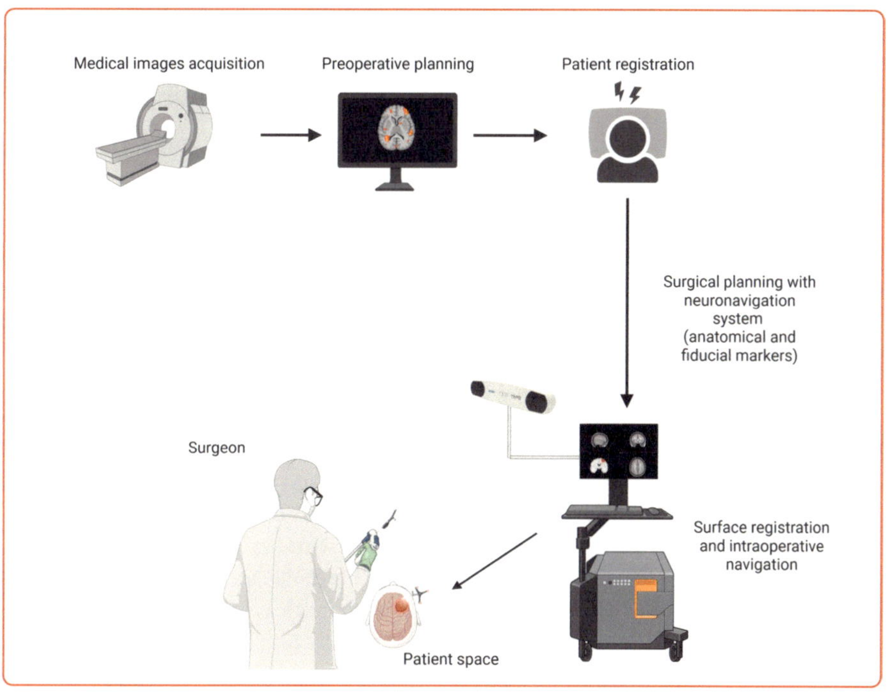

Figure 2.
Application of neuronavigation in a neurosurgical context. Operational view of a neuronavigation system used during a neurosurgical procedure. The platform provides real-time intraoperative visualization of brain structures, enhancing accuracy in tumor resection, epilepsy surgery, and functional neurosurgery.

healthy brain tissue responsible for neurocognitive function [1, 10, 33–34, 58]. Neuronavigation systems display real-time imaging data, allowing the surgical team to confirm complete tumour removal and adjust intraoperative strategies accordingly [59]. In addition, the introduction and implementation of advanced neuronavigation technologies has created enhanced spatial awareness of critical neuroanatomical regions — including key motor, sensory and language areas [58]. This enables minimally invasive surgical techniques while avoiding critical areas for speech or movement, even if these regions are near the tumour. The integration of state-of-the-art imaging techniques and neuronavigation improves the accuracy of the procedures performed by experts, increasing patient safety and treatment outcomes. By incorporating preoperative MRI and CT scans, neuronavigation systems offer real-time visualisation of the tumour's location and its relation to critical brain structures. This is particularly beneficial in cases involving tumours located near the eloquent cortex or deep within the brain [60–61]. The use of intraoperative imaging modalities, such as ultrasound and intraoperative MRI, further refines neuronavigation, allowing for real-time adjustments during surgery to ensure maximal safe resection. This leads to improved patient outcomes, reduced neurological deficits, and enhanced quality of life. The use of neuronavigation has improved the success and efficiency of surgical treatment, leading to higher rates of tumour control and fewer neurological complications. Despite these advances, challenges remain, particularly in addressing measurement inaccuracies associated with factors such as brain displacement, swelling, haemorrhage and patient movement. These factors can significantly affect the quality of imaging and the accuracy of navigation during complicated surgical procedures. Future advances in neuronavigation should focus on mitigating these inaccuracies to maximise the benefits of the technology. Improvements in surgical practise must prioritise patient outcomes by using state-of-the-art technologies to advance medicine and surgery. Continuous innovation in neuronavigation is critical to achieving these goals.

4.2 Epilepsy surgery

The increasing use of visual technology is now a cornerstone of the surgical treatment of epilepsy, as it makes the localisation and removal of the epileptogenic zone even more precise. A surgical strategy is not just another item on the treatment menu but is often the last resort for those patients whose seizures have not responded to multiple medications. With such complex surgical techniques, it is important to precisely define the location of the epileptic focus. The integration of these approaches with neuronavigation in the surgical planning phase should be considered standard practice [62]. In addition, frameless stereotactic neuronavigation improves the precision of localisation of the epileptogenic focus [63].

The CyberKnife system, for example, is a state-of-the-art robotic radiosurgery platform that combines CT and MRI information to precisely deliver ionising radiation to brain lesions [63]. The principles of neuronavigation are crucial for the precise targeting of these lesions with CyberKnife. This targeted procedure offers a non-invasive alternative to conventional surgery. By improving visualisation and planning capabilities, these advanced techniques optimise the effectiveness and safety of epilepsy surgery, allowing surgeons to precisely locate seizure foci while reducing damage to critical brain regions [63].

5. Usage protocols

The effective use of neuronavigation requires a precisely defined protocol:

- *Image acquisition*: neuroimaging (MRI, CT, PET) is performed according to specific protocols for the surgical procedure. It is crucial to minimise artefacts and obtain high quality images.

- *Preoperative planning*: Using neuronavigation software, the surgeon defines the surgical target, the access routes and the structures to be avoided. Planning can include segmentation of tumours, definition of brain nuclei for DBS or mapping of eloquent areas using fMRI.

- *Patient registration*: Registration matches the space of the preoperative images with the physical space of the patient. This can be done as follows:

- *Anatomical landmarks*: Identification of anatomical points that are easily recognisable both on the images and on the patient (e.g. the outer canthus of the eye and the root of the nose).

- *Fiducial markers*: Radiopaque markers are applied to the patient's head before the image is taken. These markers are easily recognisable both on the images and during registration.

- *Surface registration*: Use of a scanner or probe to capture a point cloud on the surface of the patient's head, which is then compared with a surface reconstructed from the preoperative images.

- *Instrument calibration*: Surgical instruments are calibrated to determine their position relative to the tracking markers or sensors.

- *Intraoperative navigation*: During the procedure, the neuronavigation system displays the position of the instruments in real time on the preoperative images so that the surgeon can navigate precisely to the target.

- *Postoperative verification*: Postoperative images (CT and MRI) can be acquired to verify the correct positioning of the instruments or the extent of the resection.

5.1 Workflow for DBS

1. Preoperative planning:

   a. *Imaging:* High-resolution MRI (T1-weighted, T2-weighted) to visualise the target nuclei (e.g. the subthalamic nucleus and the globus pallidus internus). Sometimes a CT scan is also used to plan the transcranial approach.

   b. *Segmentation:* The target nuclei are segmented manually or automatically on the MRI images.

c. *Trajectory planning:* The electrode path is planned to avoid vascular and ventricular structures and to reach the target at an optimal angle. Specialised software is often used for DBS planning.

d. *Integration of fMRI* (if applicable): If the patient has undergone task-based fMRI to map motor or cognitive function, this data is integrated into the planning to avoid critical functional areas during electrode placement.

2. Surgical procedure:

a. *Registration*: The patient is registered with the neuronavigation system using fiducial markers or anatomical landmarks.

b. *Electrode implantation*: A small burr hole is created and the DBS electrode is advanced along the planned trajectory using the neuronavigation system for real-time guidance.

c. *Microelectrode recording* (optional): Microelectrode recording can be used to further refine electrode placement based on the characteristic electrophysiological activity of the target structure.

d. *Intraoperative stimulation* (optional): Intraoperative stimulation can be performed to assess the clinical effects and identify any side effects.

3. Postoperative verification:

a. *Imaging*: postoperative CT to verify the position of the electrode.

b. *Programming*: The electrode is programmed to ensure optimal stimulation and reduce side effects. Programming is an iterative process that requires long-term follow-up.

5.2 Workflow for TMS

1. Pretreatment planning:

a. *Imaging:* High-resolution, high-resolution T1-weighted MRI may be performed to provide an anatomical reference for target localisation. While not always mandatory, it significantly enhances the accuracy of the targeting process.

b. *Integration of fMRI* (if applicable): Functional MRI may be used to map cortical targets, utilising task-related activity and resting state connectivity. This is particularly useful for setting personalised treatment goals.

c. *Data loading:* The MRI and fMRI data are loaded into the neuronavigation system to facilitate target localisation.

d. *Coordinate calculation*: The neuronavigation system computes the coordinates, often utilising MNI or Talairach spaces, to pinpoint the target accurately.

2. Registration of the patient:

 a. *Patient positioning:* The patient is seated comfortably, and the TMS coil is positioned above their head.

 b. *Head registration:* The patient's head is registered using the MRI data. Anatomical landmarks such as the nasion, inion, and preauricular points are employed to align the head with the MRI model.

 c. *Surface matching:* A 3D camera scans the patient's head, and an infrared tracking system is used to match the scanned surface to the MRI model.

 d. *Tracking of coil position:* The neuronavigation system tracks both the position and orientation of the coil relative to the target throughout the procedure.

 e. *Motorised threshold determination:* TMS is only initiated after determining the resting motor threshold (rMT). The motor cortex is stimulated, typically in the hand area, to identify the minimal stimulus required to induce a visible muscle twitch in the contralateral hand. The rMT serves as the baseline for adjusting stimulation intensity in subsequent therapeutic sessions.

3. TMS stimulation:

 a. *Coil positioning:* The TMS coil is positioned over the identified target region, and its placement is monitored in real-time with the neuronavigation system to ensure optimal positioning.

 b. *Stimulation parameters:* The stimulation parameters, such as frequency, intensity (relative to rMT), pulse pattern, number of pulses, and interval between sessions, are set according to established protocols while considering individual patient characteristics.

 c. *Administration of pulses:* The neuronavigation system ensures the accuracy of the coil placement during each stimulation pulse, which is continuously maintained throughout the session.

4. Post-treatment verification:

 a. *Response monitoring:* The patient's response to the stimulation is continuously monitored throughout the session, with adjustments made to the coil's position and stimulation parameters as necessary to optimise the therapeutic effect and minimise discomfort.

 b. *Safety monitoring:* The scalp temperature is monitored to prevent overheating, and the patient is observed for any adverse effects during the procedure.

5.3 Workflow for tumour resection

1. Preoperative Planning:

 a. *Imaging*: MRI with and without contrast, DTI (Diffusion Tensor Imaging) to visualise the tumour and surrounding structures (eloquent areas, white matter tracts).

b. *Segmentation*: The tumour and critical structures are segmented on the MRI images.

c. *Integration of fMRI*: Task-based fMRI is used to identify and map eloquent areas (motor, sensory, language) near the tumour. This data is then integrated into the neuronavigation system to guide surgical planning and minimise the risk of postoperative deficits.

d. *Resection Planning*: The resection strategy is defined to maximise tumour removal and minimise the risk of neurological deficits.

2. Surgical Procedure:

a. *Registration*: The patient is registered to the neuronavigation system using fiducial markers or anatomical landmarks.

b. *Guidance during Resection*: During resection, the neuronavigation system displays the position of the surgical instruments relative to the tumour and critical structures, allowing the surgeon to navigate precisely.

c. *Intraoperative Imaging* (Optional): Intraoperative ultrasound or MRI can be used to evaluate the extent of resection in real time and to identify any residual tumour.

3. Postoperative Verification:

a. *Imaging*: Postoperative MRI to evaluate the extent of resection and identify any complications.

6. Challenges and future directions

Neuronavigation will continue to evolve through the integration of artificial intelligence (AI), machine learning (ML) and augmented/virtual reality (AR/VR) technologies [64]. These innovations have the potential to increase surgical precision, streamline workflows and improve patient outcomes. However, to fully realise the potential of these technologies, several challenges need to be overcome.

The integration of AI and ML algorithms into neuronavigation systems can facilitate real-time image analysis, predictive modelling and personalised surgical planning. AI-powered tools can automatically segment brain structures, identify critical functional areas and predict the optimal surgical approach based on the patient's individual anatomy and pathology. However, concerns regarding data privacy, algorithmic bias and regulatory approvals must be carefully considered.

AR/VR technologies offer new opportunities for surgical education, preoperative planning and intraoperative guidance [65]. AR overlays can provide surgeons with real-time information about the anatomy and function of the brain, improving spatial awareness and surgical precision [65]. VR simulations can allow surgeons to practise complex procedures in a safe and controlled environment, improving their surgical skills and reducing the risk of complications [65]. However, developing user-friendly interfaces and validating the effectiveness of these technologies in clinical practise is still a challenge.

DOI: http://dx.doi.org/10.5772/intechopen.1010245

Overcoming these challenges will require a collaborative effort between neurosurgeons, engineers, data scientists and regulators. The application of neuronavigation in neuromodulation extends beyond TMS and DBS, with growing interest in its role in real-time functional monitoring networks [47–49]. Evidence form recent studies suggest that combining neuronavigated neurostimulation with behavioural interventions could enhance cognitive and affective outcomes, paving the way for novel multimodal therapeutic strategies [47–49]. By embracing innovation while carefully considering the ethical and practical implications, we can realise the full potential of neuronavigation and transform neurosurgical care.

7. Conclusions

Neuronavigation has fundamentally reshaped modern neurosurgery, enabling more precise and less invasive interventions across a spectrum of neurological and psychiatric conditions. By integrating advanced neuroimaging techniques with real-time surgical navigation, neuronavigation enhances the accuracy of tumour resection, optimises electrode placement in neuromodulation procedures, and facilitates the identification of epileptogenic zones in epilepsy surgery.

The ongoing integration of artificial intelligence, machine learning, and augmented/virtual reality technologies holds immense promise for further advancing the field. These innovations have the potential to refine surgical planning, automate image analysis, and provide surgeons with immersive training and guidance. However, realising the full potential of these technologies requires addressing challenges related to data privacy, algorithmic bias, and standardisation of protocols.

Despite these challenges, the future of neuronavigation is bright. By fostering collaboration among neurosurgeons, engineers, data scientists, and regulatory agencies, we can continue to push the boundaries of what is possible and improve the lives of patients with neurological and psychiatric disorders.

Conflict of interest

The authors declare no conflict of interest.

Author details

Chiara Di Fazio[1,2] and Sara Palermo[2,3,4]*

1 International School of Advanced Studies, University of Camerino, Camerino, Italy

2 Department of Psychology, University of Turin, Turin, Italy

3 Neuroscience Institute of Turin (NIT), Turin, Italy

4 Neuroradiology Unit, Diagnostic and Technology Department, "Institute of Scientific Hospitalization and Care" Foundation (IRCCS), Neurological Institute "Carlo Besta", Milan, Italy

*Address all correspondence to: sara.palermo@unito.it

References

[1] Orringer DA, Golby A, Jolesz F. Neuronavigation in the surgical management of brain tumors: Current and future trends. Expert Review of Medical Devices. 2012;**9**(5):491-500. DOI: 10.1586/erd.12.42

[2] Yen C, Lin CL, Chiang MC. Exploring the Frontiers of neuroimaging: A review of recent advances in understanding brain functioning and disorders. Life (Basel). 2023;**13**(7):1472. DOI: 10.3390/life13071472

[3] Ogando-Rivas E, Castillo P, Beltran JQ, Arellano R, Galvan-Remigio I, Soto-Ulloa V, et al. Evolution and revolution of imaging Technologies in Neurosurgery. Neurologia Medico-Chirurgica (Tokyo). 2022;**62**(12):542-551. DOI: 10.2176/jns-nmc.2022-0116

[4] Hayhurst C, Byrne P, Eldridge PR, Mallucci CL. Application of electromagnetic technology to neuronavigation: A revolution in image-guided neurosurgery. Journal of Neurosurgery. 2009;**111**(6):1179-1184. DOI: 10.3171/2008.12.JNS08628

[5] Keeble H, Lavrador JP, Pereira N, Lente K, Brogna C, Gullan R, et al. Electromagnetic navigation systems and intraoperative neuromonitoring: Reliability and feasibility study. Operative Neurosurgery (Hagerstown). 2021;**20**(4):373-382. DOI: 10.1093/ons/opaa407

[6] Tanaka S, Puffer RC, Hoover JM, Goerss SJ, Haugen LM, McGee K, et al. Increased frameless stereotactic accuracy with high-field intraoperative magnetic resonance imaging. Neurosurgery. 2012;**71**(2 Suppl. Operative):ons321-8. DOI: 10.1227/NEU.0b013e31826a88a9

[7] Kekhia H, Rigolo L, Norton I, Golby AJ. Special surgical considerations for functional brain mapping. Neurosurgery Clinics of North America. 2011;**22**(2):111-vii. DOI: 10.1016/j.nec.2011.01.004

[8] Anderson IA, Chumas PD. Neuronavigation as a diagnostic tool: An innovative application. British Journal of Neurosurgery. 2016;**30**(3):351-352. DOI: 10.3109/02688697.2015.1119239

[9] Krüger MT, Várkuti B, Achinger J, Coenen VA, Prokop T, Delev D, et al. Navigated deep brain stimulation surgery: Evaluating the combined use of a frame-based stereotactic system and a navigation system. Stereotactic and Functional Neurosurgery. 2021;**99**(1):48-54. DOI: 10.1159/000510528

[10] Lakhani DA, Sabsevitz DS, Chaichana KL, Quiñones-Hinojosa A, Middlebrooks EH. Current state of functional MRI in the presurgical planning of brain tumors. Radiology: Imaging Cancer. 2023;**5**(6):e230078. DOI: 10.1148/rycan.230078

[11] Dong Z, Andrews T, Xie C, Yokoo T. Advances in MRI techniques and applications. BioMed Research International. 2015;**2015**:139043. DOI: 10.1155/2015/139043

[12] Yousaf T, Dervenoulas G, Politis M. Advances in MRI methodology. International Review of Neurobiology. 2018;**141**:31-76. DOI: 10.1016/bs.irn.2018.08.008

[13] Hespel AM, Cole RC. Advances in high-field MRI. The Veterinary Clinics of North America. Small Animal Practice. 2018;**48**(1):11-29. DOI: 10.1016/j.cvsm.2017.08.002

[14] Harisinghani MG, O'Shea A, Weissleder R. Advances in clinical MRI technology. Science Translational Medicine. 2019;**11**(523):eaba2591. DOI: 10.1126/scitranslmed.aba2591

[15] Liu TT. MRI in systems medicine. Wiley Interdisciplinary Reviews. Systems Biology and Medicine. 2020;**12**(1):e1463. DOI: 10.1002/wsbm.1463

[16] Zhou Y, Wang H, Liu C, Liao B, Li Y, Zhu Y, et al. Recent advances in highly accelerated 3D MRI. Physics in Medicine and Biology. 2023;**68**(14):1-27. DOI: 10.1088/1361-6560/acc0cd

[17] Moglia T, Falkenstein C, Rieker F, Tun N, Rajaram-Gilkes M. Anatomical ignorance resulting in iatrogenic causes of human morbidity. Cureus. 2024;**16**(3):e56480. DOI: 10.7759/cureus.56480

[18] Slavin KV. Neuronavigation in neurosurgery: Current state of affairs. Expert Review of Medical Devices. 2008;**5**(1):1-3. DOI: 10.1586/17434440.5.1.1

[19] Ivanov M, Ciurea AV. Neuronavigation. Principles. Surgical technique. Journal of Medicine and Life. 2009;**2**(1):29-35

[20] Hayhurst C, Byrne P, Eldridge PR, Mallucci CL. Application of electromagnetic technology to neuronavigation: A revolution in image-guided neurosurgery. Journal of Neurosurgery. 2009;**111**(6):1179-1184. DOI: 10.3171/2008.12.JNS08628

[21] Stieglitz LH, Raabe A, Beck J. Simple accuracy enhancing techniques in neuronavigation. World Neurosurgery. 2015;**84**(2):580-584. DOI: 10.1016/j.wneu.2015.03.025

[22] Chartrain AG, Kellner CP, Fargen KM, Spiotta AM, Chesler DA, Fiorella D, et al. A review and comparison of three neuronavigation systems for minimally invasive intracerebral hemorrhage evacuation. Journal of Neurointerventional Surgery. 2018;**10**(1):66-74. DOI: 10.1136/neurintsurg-2017-013091

[23] Brahme A, Nyman P, Skatt B. 4D laser camera for accurate patient positioning, collision avoidance, image fusion and adaptive approaches during diagnostic and therapeutic procedures. Medical Physics. 2008;**35**(5):1670-1681. DOI: 10.1118/1.2889720

[24] Drouin S, Kochanowska A, Kersten-Oertel M, Gerard IJ, Zelmann R, De Nigris D, et al. IBIS: An OR ready open-source platform for image-guided neurosurgery. International Journal of Computer Assisted Radiology and Surgery. 2017;**12**(3):363-378. DOI: 10.1007/s11548-016-1478-0

[25] Yavas G, Caliskan KE, Cagli MS. Three-dimensional-printed marker-based augmented reality neuronavigation: A new neuronavigation technique. Neurosurgical Focus. 2021;**51**(2):E20. DOI: 10.3171/2021.5.FOCUS21206

[26] Faraj MK, Kailan SL, Al-Neami AQH. A new simple, cost-effective navigation system (EASY navigator) for neurosurgical interventions. World Neurosurgery. 2022;**164**:143-147. DOI: 10.1016/j.wneu.2022.04.100

[27] Markl M, Schnell S, Wu C, Bollache E, Jarvis K, Barker AJ, et al. Advanced flow MRI: Emerging techniques and applications. Clinical Radiology. 2016;**71**(8):779-795. DOI: 10.1016/j.crad.2016.01.011

[28] Schnell S, Wu C, Ansari SA. Four-dimensional MRI flow examinations in cerebral and extracerebral vessels - Ready for clinical routine? Current Opinion in Neurology. 2016;**29**(4):419-428. DOI: 10.1097/WCO.0000000000000341

[29] Brett M, Johnsrude IS, Owen AM. The problem of functional localization in the human brain. Nature Reviews. Neuroscience. 2002;**3**(3):243-249. DOI: 10.1038/nrn756

[30] Raichle ME. Functional brain imaging and human brain function. The Journal of Neuroscience. 2003;**23**(10):3959-3962. DOI: 10.1523/JNEUROSCI.23-10-03959.2003

[31] Lauritzen M, Gold L. Brain function and neurophysiological correlates of signals used in functional neuroimaging. The Journal of Neuroscience. 2003;**23**(10):3972-3980. DOI: 10.1523/JNEUROSCI.23-10-03972.2003

[32] Oishi M, Uzuka T, Yoneoka Y, Fujii Y, Igarashi H. New diagnostic imaging methods in neurosurgery: Advent of anatomical and functional neuroimaging. No Shinkei Geka. 2007;**35**(3):291-300

[33] Villanueva-Meyer JE, Mabray MC, Cha S. Current clinical brain tumor imaging. Neurosurgery. 2017;**81**(3):397-415. DOI: 10.1093/neuros/nyx103

[34] Sabeghi P, Zarand P, Zargham S, Golestany B, Shariat A, Chang M, et al. Advances in neuro-oncological imaging: An update on diagnostic approach to brain tumors. Cancers (Basel). 2024;**16**(3):576. DOI: 10.3390/cancers16030576

[35] Pelletier I, Sauerwein HC, Lepore F, Saint-Amour D, Lassonde M. Non-invasive alternatives to the Wada test in the presurgical evaluation of language and memory functions in epilepsy patients. Epileptic Disorders. 2007;**9**(2):111-126. DOI: 10.1684/epd.2007.0109

[36] Lee MH, Smyser CD, Shimony JS. Resting-state fMRI: A review of methods and clinical applications. AJNR. American Journal of Neuroradiology. 2013;**34**(10):1866-1872. DOI: 10.3174/ajnr.A3263

[37] Lee MH, Miller-Thomas MM, Benzinger TL, Marcus DS, Hacker CD, Leuthardt EC, et al. Clinical resting-state fMRI in the preoperative setting: Are we ready for prime time? Topics in Magnetic Resonance Imaging. 2016;**25**(1):11-18. DOI: 10.1097/RMR.0000000000000075

[38] Hacker CD, Roland JL, Kim AH, Shimony JS, Leuthardt EC. Resting-state network mapping in neurosurgical practice: A review. Neurosurgical Focus. 2019;**47**(6):E15. DOI: 10.3171/2019.9.FOCUS19656

[39] Abrantes AM, Pires AS, Monteiro L, Teixo R, Neves AR, Tavares NT, et al. Tumour functional imaging by PET. Biochimica et Biophysica Acta - Molecular Basis of Disease. 2020;**1866**(6):165717. DOI: 10.1016/j.bbadis.2020.165717

[40] Yan Q, Yan X, Yang X, et al. The use of PET/MRI in radiotherapy. Insights Into Imaging. 2024;**15**:63. DOI: 10.1186/s13244-024-01627-6

[41] Lozano AM, Lipsman N, Bergman H, Brown P, Chabardes S, Chang JW, et al. Deep brain stimulation: Current challenges and future directions. Nature Reviews. Neurology. 2019;**15**(3):148-160. DOI: 10.1038/s41582-018-0128-2

[42] Krauss JK, Lipsman N, Aziz T, Boutet A, Brown P, Chang JW, et al. Technology of deep brain stimulation: Current status and future directions.

Nature Reviews. Neurology. 2021;**17**(2):75-87. DOI: 10.1038/s41582-020-00426-z

[43] Bjartmarz H, Rehncrona S. Comparison of accuracy and precision between frame-based and frameless stereotactic navigation for deep brain stimulation electrode implantation. Stereotactic and Functional Neurosurgery. 2007;**85**(5):235-242. DOI: 10.1159/000103262

[44] Krüger MT, Várkuti B, Achinger J, Coenen VA, Prokop T, Delev D, et al. Navigated deep brain stimulation surgery: Evaluating the combined use of a frame-based stereotactic system and a navigation system. Stereotactic and Functional Neurosurgery. 2021;**99**(1):48-54. DOI: 10.1159/000510528

[45] Di Fazio C, Palermo S. Aging pathways: Unraveling geriatric neuropsychology and innovative neuromodulatory treatments in the new millennium. In: Advances in Geriatrics and Gerontology - Challenges of the New Millennium. London, UK: IntechOpen; 2024. DOI: 10.5772/intechopen.114842

[46] Zhong G, Yang Z, Jiang T. Precise modulation strategies for transcranial magnetic stimulation: Advances and future directions. Neuroscience Bulletin. 2021;**37**(12):1718-1734. DOI: 10.1007/s12264-021-00781-x

[47] Palermo S, Di Fazio C, Scaliti E, Stanziano M, Nigri A, Tamietto M. Cortical excitability and the aging brain: Toward a biomarker of cognitive resilience. Frontiers in Psychology. 2025;**16**:1542880. DOI: 10.3389/fpsyg.2025.1542880

[48] Di Fazio C, Tamietto M, Stanziano M, Nigri A, Scaliti E, Palermo S. Cortico–cortical paired associative stimulation (ccPAS) in ageing and Alzheimer's disease: A quali-quantitative approach to potential therapeutic mechanisms and applications. Brain Sciences. 2025;**15**(3):237. DOI: 10.3390/brainsci15030237

[49] Di Fazio C, Scaliti E, Stanziano M, Nigri A, De Michelis G, Tamietto M, et al. Rewiring the aging brain: The impact of rTMS on cognitive function and mood. Brain Stimulation. 2025;**18**(1):372. DOI: 10.1016/j.brs.2024.12.473

[50] Isaacs BR, Heijmans M, Kuijf ML, Kubben PL, Ackermans L, Temel Y, et al. Variability in subthalamic nucleus targeting for deep brain stimulation with 3 and 7 tesla magnetic resonance imaging. NeuroImage Clinical. 2021;**32**:102829. DOI: 10.1016/j.nicl.2021.102829

[51] Rao AT, Chou KL, Patil PG. Localization of deep brain stimulation trajectories via automatic mapping of microelectrode recordings to MRI. Journal of Neural Engineering. 2023;**20**(1):1-14. DOI: 10.1088/1741-2552/acbb2b

[52] Muthuraman M, Chirumamilla CV, Groppa S. Establishing standards for neuronavigated TMS in research and clinical studies. Clinical Neurophysiology. 2016;**127**(8):2890-2891. DOI: 10.1016/j.clinph.2016.05.009

[53] Siebner HR, Funke K, Aberra AS, Antal A, Bestmann S, Chen R, et al. Transcranial magnetic stimulation of the brain: What is stimulated? - a consensus and critical position paper. Clinical Neurophysiology. 2022;**140**:59-97. DOI: 10.1016/j.clinph.2022.04.022

[54] Sun W, Wu Q, Gao L, Zheng Z, Xiang H, Yang K, et al. Advancements in transcranial magnetic stimulation

research and the path to precision. Neuropsychiatric Disease and Treatment. 2023;**19**:1841-1851. DOI: 10.2147/NDT.S414782

[55] Tikka SK, Siddiqui MA, Garg S, Pattojoshi A, Gautam M. Clinical practice guidelines for the therapeutic use of repetitive transcranial magnetic stimulation in neuropsychiatric disorders. Indian Journal of Psychiatry. 2023;**65**(2):270-288. DOI: 10.4103/indianjpsychiatry.indianjpsychiatry_492_22

[56] Jolesz FA. MRI-guided focused ultrasound surgery. Annual Review of Medicine. 2009;**60**:417-430. DOI: 10.1146/annurev.med.60.041707.170303

[57] Stanziano M, Golfrè Andreasi N, Messina G, Rinaldo S, Palermo S, Verri M, et al. Resting state functional connectivity signatures of MRgFUS vim thalamotomy in Parkinson's disease: A preliminary study. Frontiers in Neurology. 2022;**12**:786734. DOI: 10.3389/fneur.2021.786734

[58] Perera Valdivia D, Zapata Vega L, Herrera Pérez E, Toledo Cisneros F, Gómez López L, Guzmán Reynoso L, et al. Effects of the use of neuronavigation in patients with supratentorial brain gliomas: A cohort study. World Neurosurgery. 2024;**187**:e860-e869. DOI: 10.1016/j.wneu.2024.05.002

[59] Sulangi AJ, Husain A, Lei H, Okun J. Neuronavigation in glioma resection: Current applications, challenges, and clinical outcomes. Frontiers in Surgery. 2024;**11**:1430567. DOI: 10.3389/fsurg.2024.1430567

[60] Kumar A, Chandra PS, Sharma BS, Garg A, Rath GK, Bithal PK, et al. The role of neuronavigation-guided functional MRI and diffusion tensor tractography along with cortical stimulation in patients with eloquent cortex lesions. British Journal of Neurosurgery. 2014;**28**(2):226-233. DOI: 10.3109/02688697.2013.835370

[61] Hassan MA, Shah SA, Rehman RAU, Yasir MU, Khan AYR, Qureshi MN, et al. Role of neuro navigation in enhancing surgical precision: A single-center experience – A comprehensive review article. Journal of Health and Rehabilitation Research. 2024;**4**(1):1239-1242. DOI: 10.61919/jhrr.v4i1.591

[62] Stone SS, Rutka JT. Utility of neuronavigation and neuromonitoring in epilepsy surgery. Neurosurgical Focus. 2008;**25**(3):E17. DOI: 10.3171/FOC/2008/25/9/E17

[63] Cheng Y, Lin Y, Long Y, Du L, Chen R, Hu T, et al. Is the CyberKnife© radiosurgery system effective and safe for patients? An umbrella review of the evidence. Future Oncology. 2022;**18**(14):1777-1791. DOI: 10.2217/fon-2021-0844

[64] Kazemzadeh K, Akhlaghdoust M, Zali A. Advances in artificial intelligence, robotics, augmented and virtual reality in neurosurgery. Frontiers in Surgery. 2023;**10**:1241923. DOI: 10.3389/fsurg.2023.1241923

[65] Cho J, Rahimpour S, Cutler A, Goodwin CR, Lad SP, Codd P. Enhancing reality: A systematic review of augmented reality in neuronavigation and education. World Neurosurgery. 2020;**139**:186-195. DOI: 10.1016/j.wneu.2020.04.043